LB01095

D0597150

HEALTH CAREERS / PTAT

REHABILITATION
of the
BURN PATIENT

CLINICS IN PHYSICAL THERAPY
VOLUME 4

EDITORIAL BOARD

Otto D. Payton, Ph.D., **Chairman**

Louis R. Amundsen, Ph.D.

Suzann K. Campbell, Ph.D.

Jules M. Rothstein, Ph.D.

Shirley Sahrmann, Ph.D.

Steven L. Wolf, Ph.D.

REHABILITATION
of the
BURN PATIENT

Edited by

Vincent R. DiGregorio, M.D.

Associate Director, Burn Center
Nassau County Medical Center
East Meadow, New York
Chief, Section of Plastic Surgery
Nassau Hospital
Mineola, New York

CHURCHILL LIVINGSTONE

NEW YORK, EDINBURGH, LONDON, AND MELBOURNE

1984

Acquisitions editor: William R. Schmitt
Copy editor: Steven B. Levy
Production editor: Michiko Davis
Production supervisor: Sharon Tuder
Composition: The Maple-Vail Book Manufacturing Group
Printer/Binder: The Maple Press Company

© Churchill Livingstone Inc. 1984

All rights reserved. No part of this publication may be reproduced,
stored in a retrieval system, or transmitted in any form or by any
means, electronic, mechanical, photocopying, recording or otherwise,
without prior permission of the publishers (Churchill Livingstone
Inc., 1560 Broadway, New York, N.Y. 10036).

Distributed in the United Kingdom by Churchill Livingstone, Robert
Stevenson House, 1–3 Baxter's Place, Leith Walk, Edinburgh EH1
3AF and by associated companies, branches and representatives
throughout the world.

First published 1984
Printed in U.S.A.

ISBN 0-443-08200-6
7 6 5 4 3 2 1

Library of Congress Cataloging in Publication Data
Main entry under title:

Rehabilitation of the burn patient.

   (Clinics in physical therapy; v. 4)
   Bibliography: p.
   Includes index.
   1. Burns and scalds—Patients—Rehabilitation.
I. DiGregorio, Vincent R. II. Series.
RD96.4.R44 1984   617'.1106   83-15239
ISBN 0-443-08200-6

Manufactured in the United States of America

To my father, Nicholas John DiGregorio, M.D.,
who has been a constant source of
inspiration to my career and life

Contributors

Vincent R. DiGregorio, M.D.
Associate Director, Burn Center, Nassau County Medical Center, East Meadow, New York; Chief, Section of Plastic Surgery, Nassau Hospital, Mineola, New York

Nora Goldberg, O.T.R.
Occupational Therapist, Long Island College Hospital, Brooklyn, New York

Nancy Newton Hanson, R.P.T.
Chief Physical Therapist (Former), Shriners Burns Institute, Boston, Massachusetts

Julianne W. Howell, R.P.T.
Wishard Memorial Hospital, Department of Rehabilitation Medicine, Indiana University Medical Center, Indianapolis, Indiana

Mitch Kaplan, M.D.
Department of Plastic Surgery, Long Island College Hospital, Brooklyn, New York

Patricia M. Kozerefski, R.P.T.
Assistant Chief Physical Therapist, Supervisor of Rehabilitation Services for Burn Center, The New York Hospital–Cornell Medical Center, New York, New York

Jean LeMaster, L.P.T.
Senior Physical Therapist, University of Iowa Hospitals and Clinics, Clinical Instructor, Physical Therapy Education, University of Iowa, Iowa City, Iowa

Irwin E. Mendelsohn, M.D., F.A.P.M., F.A.A.P.
Attending Psychiatrist, Consultant (Psychiatric) to the Burn Center, Nassau County Medical Center, East Meadow, New York; Assistant Clinical Professor of Psychiatry, School of Medicine, State University of New York at Stony Brook, Stony Brook, New York

Patti Stadler, O.T.
Occupational Therapist, Nassau County Medical Center, East Meadow, New York

Linda J. Zane, R.P.T.
Assistant Chief Physical Therapist, Nassau County Medical Center, East Meadow, New York

Preface

Physical therapists and occupational therapists are some of the more important and active members of the burn team. As therapists gain more experience in the treatment of burn patients, their contributions and responsibilities increase rapidly. Depending upon the characteristics of the burn treatment facility, the therapists are now routinely initiating and performing procedures that were previously outside the realm of classical training. Because of the amount of time spent with the patient and because of the intimate relationship that develops during the prolonged hospital stay, the therapist may be the burn team member with whom the burn victim identifies most closely. In addition, unlike some of the other members of the burn team, because of the prolonged rehabilitative process the relationship usually extends well beyond the initial hospitalization.

This book was written because of a very real need for its existence and because of the gap in burn treatment education which exists in the traditional physical therapy and occupational therapy curriculum. Unfortunately, many physical therapist and occupational therapist training programs are not associated with one of the very few specialized burn treatment facilities that exist. This volume will provide basic information for those therapists who are first coming into contact with the burn patient, and it will prove to be a valuable resource for those therapists who see the occasional burn patient.

This volume is not a cookbook manual but a text which explains the physiological and pathological basis for managing acutely ill burn patients. A thorough understanding of these factors allows for more appropriately planned and timed therapy. It can be read in its entirety as a text for the student or experienced practitioner unfamiliar with the burn patient, or it can be used as a reference resource for the burn therapist having a specific problem with an unusual circumstance.

Vincent R. DiGregorio, M.D.

Contents

REHABILITATION
of the
BURN PATIENT

1 | The Burn Problem, the Burn Team, and the Physical Therapist

Vincent R. DiGregorio

THE BURN PROBLEM

It is very difficult to estimate the magnitude of the problem of burn care management in the United States; however, by examining some of the newly generated burn statistics, we can get some feeling for the dimensions of the problem. It has been estimated that 2,500,000 people in the United States suffer burn wounds annually, resulting in at least 12,000 deaths.[1] Of course, millions of patients are not treated at the small number of burn treatment facilities available in this country; the majority of these patients are treated as outpatients. Unfortunately, there are no statistics available that would tell us the number of patients treated at specific burn treatment centers annually. We shall be concerned in this book with those patients who suffer major burns, are hospitalized, and come into the care of a physical therapist, either as inpatients or outpatients.

According to the classification established by the American Burn Association, major burns that are usually treated in specialized burn treatment centers are classified as follows:

1. second-degree burns of 25 percent or greater total body surface area in adults, or 20 percent in children.
2. third-degree burns of 10 percent or greater total body surface area.
3. burns involving specialized areas; that is, burns of the hands, feet, face, eyes, ears, or perineum.
4. burns complicated by inhalation injury.

1

5. burns complicated by fractures or other major trauma.
6. high-voltage electrical burns.
7. burns occurring in poor risk groups, such as patients with significant preexisting medical problems, head injuries, cerebral vascular accidents, or psychiatric disabilities.

The care given to patients admitted to specialized burn treatment facilities is very complex and prolonged. Although the average length of stay for all surviving patients treated in such centers is 22.4 days, it is significant that the average stay for patients over 30-years old is 55.2 days.[2] This is a very long time in an intensive care type situation when one compares it with the average total hospitalization for a myocardial infarction in a 60-year old, which is 13 days,[3] and the average total hospitalization for coronary bypass surgery, which is also 13 days.[4]

THE BURN TEAM

The natural consequence of prolonged care given in specialized burn treatment centers by many different medical specialists was the development of the burn team concept. As specialized burn treatment facilities were established over the past 20 years, it became obvious that no one individual is capable of dealing expertly or efficiently with all the demands placed upon a facility by one or several critically ill burn patients. An appreciation of this multidimensional problem led to the simultaneous, spontaneous generation of the burn team principle across the United States. Diversity of the members of the burn team, which initially were treating surgeon and nursing personnel, expanded rapidly as the level of sophistication of burn care increased. Presently the burn team usually consists of physicians and nursing personnel and additionally, a physical therapist, occupational therapist, orthotist, clinical nutritionist, social worker, vocational rehabilitation counselor, and staff psychiatrist or psychologist. Obviously, depending upon the individual characteristics of the facility, other professionals may be included in the burn treatment team.

The result of the burn team approach has been the development of a mutual respect and appreciation of each burn team member's contribution to the overall care of the patient and the development of a decision-making process that relies much upon the input of all team members. Discussions at burn team conferences not only lead to improved individual patient care, but produce a solidarity amongst team members and also provide an opportunity for members to gain insight into problems other team members have in dealing with the same patient.

THE PHYSICAL THERAPIST AND THE BURN TEAM

The physical therapist is one of the more important and active members of the burn team. As physical therapists gain more experience in the treatment of burn patients, their contributions and responsibilities increase rapidly. Again, depending upon the characteristics of the burn treatment facility, physical therapists are now routinely initiating and performing procedures that were previously outside of the realm of classical physical therapy training. Because of the amount of time spent with the patient and because of the intimate relationship that develops during the prolonged hospital stay, the physical therapist may be the burn team member with whom the burn victim identifies most closely. In addition, unlike some of the other members of the burn team, because of the prolonged rehabilitative process, the relationship usually extends well after the initial hospitalization.

PROBLEMS FACING THE PHYSICAL THERAPIST IN THE CARE OF THE BURN PATIENT

A significant burn injury maximally stresses all body systems. Although the physical therapist must be concerned with the total physiological insult, the areas of particular concern are the skin damage and the results of this damage to underlying structures. The ultimate goal of the physical therapist in the treatment of burns should be the maintenance of maximal functional use of all remaining and reconstructed parts.

Burns have been classically described as first degree, second degree, third degree, and possibly fourth degree. A first-degree burn is of little concern to us. It represents injury to the most superficial layers of the skin and clinically presents as erythema and pain. It is a self-limited condition and is comparable to the reddened sunburn.

A second-degree burn or partial-thickness injury has traditionally been described as injury that extends into the dermis and is clinically characterized by pain and blistering. With proper custodial care, second-degree burns should reepithelialize from the surviving skin appendages, such as hair follicles and sweat and sebaceous glands. However, some deeper second-degree burns, although they do epithelialize, can produce significant morbidity in terms of fibrosis, contracture, and subsequent joint stiffness. Therefore, it is more precise to divide second-degree burns into two general categories of partial-thickness injury. Superficial partial-thickness burns heal spontaneously with little morbidity. Deep partial-thickness burns produce delayed epithelialization and significant morbidity.

Third-degree burns or full-thickness burns represent injury to all layers of the skin, including epidermis, dermis, and skin appendages. In these circumstances, the damaged skin must be replaced, usually by split-thickness skin grafts from other unburned portions of the body or from healed partial-thickness areas. Obviously, when full-thickness loss is replaced by partial thickness of skin, we cannot expect the same functional and cosmetic results.

It is at times very difficult to differentiate between partial- and full-thickness injury, especially in children. Frequently this diagnosis must be made retrospectively: if the burn wound epithelializes adequately, it is a superficial second-degree burn; if the damaged skin ultimately sloughs, it is full-thickness or third-degree burn.

The term *fourth-degree burn* is sometimes used. This refers to a burn in which structures such as tendon or bone underlying the skin are also damaged. Sometimes the term *char injury* is also used in these circumstances.

RELEVANT PATHOPHYSIOLOGY OF BURNS

The basic pathophysiological consequence of the burn injury is a loss of capillary integrity leading to edema formation, which is a result of the outpouring of protein-rich intravascular fluid into the interstitium. This process occurs at all areas of partial-thickness burns and at areas adjacent to and subjacent to full-thickness burns. As the patient frequently splints the injured part because of pain, and as a result of direct damage to the lymphatic systems, this edema fluid accumulates and persists in tissue spaces around tendons, joints, and ligaments. New collagen fibers form in this protein-rich edema fluid and eventually organize into unyielding adhesions and thickened support structures whose normal elasticity is lost.[5] The collagen fibers themselves do not contract but, with prolonged immobilization, fix the structures and produce joint and structure morbidity. It is the function of all burn team members, particularly the physical therapist, to ensure that edema fluid quickly resolves and that tendons, joint capsules, and ligaments do not become limited and functionless as a result of the burn injury.

REFERENCES

1. Baxter, CR, Marvin JA, and Curreri PW: Early management of thermal burns. Postgrad Med 55:131, 1974
2. Feller I, Tholen D, and Cornell RG: Improvements in burn care. JAMA 244:2074–2078, 1965–1979
3. Length of Stay PAS Hospitals by Diagnosis, Commission on Professional and Hospital Activity. Ann Arbor, Michigan, 1980
4. Length of Stay PAS Hospitals by Operation, Commission on Professional and Hospital Activity. Ann Arbor, Michigan, 1980
5. Beasley, RW: Hand Injuries. Philadelphia, WB Saunders, 1981

2 | Evaluation of the Acutely Ill Burn Patient

Linda J. Zane

The ultimate goal of physical therapy is to assist the patient toward maximal function. The art of physical therapy lies in selecting the appropriate treatment technique for a particular patient with a specific injury, taking into consideration the patient's limitations, assets, and goals. Only through thorough evaluation and a clear understanding of the complexities of the burn patient can this goal be met.

The purpose of this chapter is to provide the therapist with a systematic approach to the evaluation of the severely injured burn patient as well as a clear understanding of the medical procedures involved in the treatment of thermal injuries. The application of this information towards developing a basic treatment program is illustrated and discussed.

INITIAL EVALUATION

Goals of Evaluation

Burns are devastating injuries as they constitute systemic disease and psychological and physical trauma, as well as localized injury.[1] Consequently, the initial evaluation must include an assessment of the mental, physical, and functional status of the patient. The goals of the therapist's evaluation process are to determine the patient's present status, identify the rehabilitation problems, and anticipate the patient's potential problems by retrieving and assessing all of the necessary information available. Meeting these goals will enable the therapist to design and implement a comprehensive treatment program that will minimize the resultant deformities and maximize the salvaged parts.

The first task is to evaluate the immediate postinjury status of the patient. The information necessary to make this determination will include an assessment of the circumstances of the injury, the duration, type, and extent of the burn, preexisting medical and rehabilitation problems, concurrent injuries, and range of motion estimates. The patient's prior ability to adjust to stress and pain should also be obtained and considered.

Identifying the rehabilitation problems of the patient requires additional information as well as an understanding of the implications of different types of burns and their locations. For example, burns of the lower extremities may confine the patient to bed. Therefore, dangling, ambulation, or table activities will not be possible. Upper extremity burns, on the other hand, represent a different set of problems requiring a constant activity and vigilance with regard to positioning the patient to minimize edema and loss of function. Facial burns may limit the patient's ability to cooperate because of dressings over the eyes and ears. These considerations should come to mind while reviewing chart data prior to examining the patient.

The expected clinical course and approximate length of stay of the patient should be estimated initially in order to anticipate potential emotional, physiological, and rehabilitation problems. Being aware of problems such as a previously poor medical status, long immobilization due to fractures, multiple grafting sessions, and inhalation injury will help to identify potential complications. For example, if the patient has suffered full-thickness burns to the posterior trunk area, he will likely spend long periods in the prone position because of multiple grafting sessions. Immediately placing the patient in the prone position in increasing increments will make it easier for the patient to tolerate this position when the grafting sessions begin. Anticipating such problems will save the patient valuable time, effort, and anguish.

The goals outlined above can only be achieved if the therapist is conscientious in initially retrieving all available information. To fulfill these goals requires the ability to watch, listen, question, examine, and review all sources of information. All pertinent, available information must then be organized into logical, flowing programs.

Sources of Information

The sources of information available to the therapist are the medical chart, physician, nurse, patient, patient's family, and other members of the burn team. Each source should be utilized to construct an accurate and complete picture of the burn patient and an effective treatment program. The information retrieved may be maintained in an independent physical therapy record. The evaluation form illustrated in Fig. 2-1 is the form used by physical therapists rotating through the Burn Center at Nassau County Medical Center. Although the form is lengthy, it provides the therapist with a rational approach to the initial evaluation of the acutely ill burn patient. The needs of a particular institution will dictate whether this form is applicable to that specific situation. An additional form to consider is illustrated in Fig. 2-2. This diagram demonstrates the sequence of the evaluation process in its entirety.

NASSAU COUNTY MEDICAL CENTER

BURN CENTER

Physical Therapy Evaluation Form

I.   NAME:_____   DATE OF INJURY:_____

     AGE:_____   DATE OF ADMISSION:_____

     % OF BURN:_____   DATE OF EVAULATION:_____

     NEXT OF KIN:_____   OCCUPATION:_____

Partial
thickness

Full
thickness

II. TYPE OF BURN:

     Open Flame ( )   Scald ( )   Chemical ( )   Electrical ( )

     Circumstances of Injury:_____
     _____
     _____
     _____

III. VITAL SIGNS:

	Pulse	Respiration	Blood Pressure	Weight
Day 1				
Day 2				
Day 3				
Day 4				
Day 5				

Fig. 2-1. Physical therapy evaluation form.

IV. HISTORY: (Check appropriate box and describe condition)

    A. Heart ( )_____

    B. Pulmonary ( )_____

    C. Renal ( )_____

    D. Rehab. ( )_____

    E. Other ( )_____

V. MENTAL STATUS:

    A. Past _____

    B. Present _____

VI. CONCURRENT INJURIES: _____

VII. TREATMENT PLAN:

                                           Comments

    A. I.V. placement ( )_____

    B. Monitor input & output ( )_____

    C. N.P.O. ( )_____

    D. Tracheostomy ( )_____

    E. Escharotomies ( )_____

    F. Cleansing orders_____

        1. tank ( )_____

        2. shower ( )_____

        3. bedside ( )_____

    G. Debridement

        1. Mechanical ( )_____

        2. Surgical ( )_____

        3. Enzymatic ( )_____

    H. Dressings

VIII. NUTRITIONAL ASSESSMENT AND PLAN:_____

Fig. 2-1   (*Continued*).

REHABILITATION PLAN

IX.   GUIDELINES FOR POSITIONING:

AFFECTED BODY PART	DESIRED POSITION	METHOD
Neck		
Trunk		
(L) Hip		
(R) Hip		
(L) Knee		
(R) Knee		
(L) Ankle		
(R) Ankle		
(L) Shoulder		
(R) Shoulder		
(L) Elbow		
(R) Elbow		
(L) Wrist		
(R) Wrist		
(L) Digits		
(R) Digits		
(L) Thumb		
(R) Thumb		

Instructions for Positioning:_____

Additional Edema Control:_____

X. RANGE OF MOTION ASSESSMENT:_____

XI. EXERCISE AND AMBULATION PLAN:_____

XII. PULMONARY TREATMENT PLAN:_____

Fig. 2-1 (*Continued*).

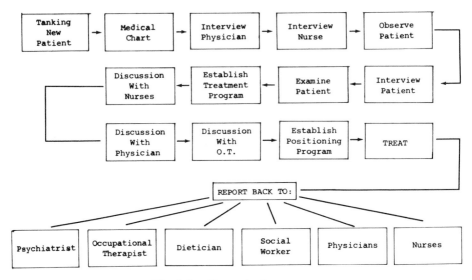

Fig. 2-2.   The evaluation process.

The first source of information to be investigated should be the patient's medical chart. Specific sections of the chart, particularly the past medical history, face sheet, burn diagram, and physician's admission note and examination, will provide a detailed account of the patient's hospital stay thus far, as well as his premorbid history and status. Other sections to be reviewed include the physician's orders and the nursing progress notes.

The medical chart should be approached in an organized fashion. Every chart will have a face sheet, which will contain the patient's name, address, age, occupation, religion, and next of kin. Obviously, different ages will present different risk factors and therapeutic problems. For example, very young and elderly patients are poor risks and may have limited ability to cooperate. The thinness of their skin often results in deeper wounds than would be expected, and their dependence on others makes treatment more difficult. In addition, the elderly burn patient is more likely to have a preexisting disease that will modify his condition and treatment.

The therapist may anticipate problems by considering the significance of the injury with regard to the occupation of the injured individual. For example, if the patient is a mailman, deep dermal burns to the lower extremities can be devastating. A secretary would be seriously affected by partial-thickness hand burns. To determine whether there is or will be a problem in this area requires an understanding of the physical, intellectual, and interpersonal requirements of the patient's job.

Following the review of the face sheet, one may then evaluate the medical history section of the chart. It will contain the physician's admission note, the burn diagram, the prior medical history, and the physical examination. The physician's admission note and physical examination will reveal the circumstances and extent of the burn, as well as any concurrent injuries. The medical history will specify any preexisting medical and rehabilitation problems. The burn diagram will illustrate which joints and body parts are involved and the estimated depth of the burn.

Knowing the type of thermal insult and the duration of exposure to that source often serves as a significant clue in assessing the severity of the burn. A knowledge of the circumstances surrounding the injury provides substantial information for differentiating between types of burns. For example, a diagnosis of an inhalation component can be ascertained by determining whether the burn was incurred in a closed space, whether there was exposure to noxious fumes, or if the patient has suffered facial burns. With a chemical burn, it is essential to know which chemical agent was involved and whether the patient was clothed over the area of injury. With an electrical burn, the type and intensity of current received can help discern the extent of injury. Moreover, the circumstances surrounding the injury should be noted, since job-related injuries and events where other individuals are killed or severely injured might affect the patient's recovery.

The physician's admission note and physical examination will document injuries incurred during the burn incident. Concurrent injuries such as open wounds, fractures, or peripheral nerve injuries will necessitate modifications and innovations in the treatment approach. For example, a recent fracture requires continuous splinting or internal fixation, which will confine the patient to bed. Furthermore, the position required to align the fracture might be contrary to the optimal position required to prevent burn wound deformities. When concurrent injuries exist, priorities need to be established and followed.

The burn diagram provides a schematic view of the extent and depth of injury. Estimates of burned area and depth are important criteria for directing resuscitation and assessing the prognosis. In addition, it has been documented that joint range of motion limitations are directly proportional to the extent of the burn.[2] The extent of healthy tissue burned or total body surface area (TBSA) involved is represented by a percentage.

At some centers, the admitting physician estimates the total percentage of burn using the Lund-Browder chart (Fig. 2-3) and sketches the burned area on the burn diagram. The Lund-Browder chart takes into consideration changes in the ratio of different body regions to the total body surface that occur with age, particularly relating to the head and lower extremities. Changes in the head, thigh, and leg are calculated at different age intervals for children, adolescents, and adults. Although initial clinical judgement of the depth of burn based on wound appearance is not always precise, the physician estimates and, using the legend on the chart, sketches the estimated depth of burn for the purposes of fluid resuscitation and transmission of information to other members of the burn team.

If the medical history reveals preexisting disease, such as cardiovascular, renal, respiratory, or metabolic disease, care will be further complicated and perhaps survival unfavorably influenced. Since the severity of a burn injury is a function of both the injury and the patient's ability to withstand it, there is wide variability in the consequences of a burn injury due to individual differences in levels of health and compliance.[3] In patients with cardiopulmonary disease, pulmonary edema is more apt to occur with the considerable replacement fluids necessary for adequate fluid resuscitation. Patients with previous arteriosclerotic disease, especially angina pectoris or past history of myocardial infarction, face the serious hazard of postburn myocardial infarction.[4] Prior renal disease exposes the patient to a greater risk of burn-associated renal failure. The additional stress and compromise to the lungs by

| | AGE (YEARS) | | | | | % | % | % |
AREA	0-1	1-4	5-9	10-15	ADULT	2	3	TOTAL
Head	19	17	13	10	7			
Neck	2	2	2	2	2			
Ant. Trunk	13	17	13	13	13			
Post. Trunk	13	13	13	13	13			
R. Buttock	2½	2½	2½	2½	2½			
L. Buttock	2½	2½	2½	2½	2½			
Genitalia	1	1	1	1	1			
R.U. Arm	4	4	4	4	4			
L.U Arm	4	4	4	4	4			
R.L. Arm	3	3	3	3	3			
L.L. Arm	3	3	3	3	3			
R. Hand	2½	2½	2½	2½	2½			
L. Hand	2½	2½	2½	2½	2½			
R. Thigh	5½	6½	8½	8½	9½			
L. Thigh	5½	6½	8½	8½	9½			
R. Leg	5	5	5½	6	7			
L. Leg	5	5	5½	6	7			
R. Foot	3½	3½	3½	3½	3½			
L. Foot	3½	3½	3½	3½	3½			
					Total			

Fig. 2-3. The Lund-Browder chart.

an inhalation injury may prove fatal to a patient with a previous respiratory disorder. Metabolic diseases, such as diabetes mellitus, predispose a patient to poor wound healing and infection.

A medical history that includes previous rehabilitation problems will necessitate modifications in treatment approach and alterations in short- and long-term goals. For example, care must be taken with arthritics so that diseased joints are not over-stressed. Obviously, in such situations, therapeutic goals must be modified. Residual spasticity or range of motion limitations from an old cerebrovascular accient (CVA) is an important consideration when administering range of motion exercises. Prior neurological deficits, such as impaired sensation, weakness, ataxia, dizziness, or pain, will call for further modifications in treatment programs. Old fractures, amputations, and congenital defects obviously require special consideration.

By judiciously evaluating the chart, the therapist may gain some idea of the expected clinical course and estimated length of stay of the patient. In addition, a picture is starting to develop as to the requirements of this particular patient necessary to ultimately insure his optimal functional level. However, further information must be retrieved from additional sources to complete the picture of the patient.

Following the medical chart evaluation, the therapist should approach the physician as a source of information. The therapist should question the physician as to his expectations of the patient's recovery and particular needs. Discuss the type of dressings, antimicrobials, surgical procedures, and debridement methods that are going to be employed. Whether the burn wounds are going to be totally covered with bulky occlusive dressings, lightly dressed with modified open technique, or left open will legislate the type of activities that can be performed and at what intervals. Whether debridement is going to be accomplished surgically, enzymatically, or mechanically will alter the treatment plan, because each method has inherent problems. Maintaining a direct line of communication with the physician on a daily basis helps to avoid confusion, determine areas of concentration, and provide for a useful source and exchange of information.

Another information source to be considered is the nursing staff, especially the head nurse or the primary nurse directly responsible for the patient. Discussion concerning the physician's orders and the scheduled treatment times are helpful. For example, dressing changes should be discussed, because it is considerably more comfortable for the patient to exercise when the dressings are removed or have been recently reapplied than to do so with dry, tight dressings. Therefore, therapy should be worked around the nurse's scheduled dressing changes. In addition, if hydrotherapy is the treatment of choice, cooperation with the nursing staff in arranging the tanking during therapy hours will help with range of motion activities.

The nurses can also provide information regarding the patient's initial psychological reaction and any information the staff has already given the patient. Understandably, burn patients and their families are emotionally labile and often express anger, grief, depression, and anxiety over seemingly minor things. It is very important that the entire staff provide structure and consistency to both the patient and family in this new alien environment.[5] Explanations of treatment procedures, schedules, and the long-term implications of a burn injury should be consistent among staff members. This will provide assurance to the patient and their family and hopefully reduce their anxiety.

After the discussion with the nursing staff, the therapist is finally ready to approach the patient, who will be the most bountiful source of information, especially for the therapist's purposes. If you were not present during the admission evaluation by the physician, try to make the first visit right before a dressing change, so that the wounds may be viewed in their entirety. Go to the patient's room and stop at the door. Resist the temptation to go immediately to the involved parts. Stand back and take a minute to view the patient as a whole. Is the patient on a respirator? Is he conscious? Does he have I.V.'s and in what locations? Is he watching TV, listening to the radio, or sleeping? The answers to these questions will help to formulate a total picture of the patient and valuable information will be gained in an indirect manner and in just a few seconds.

This is the time to establish trust and develop an ongoing relationship with the patient. Following the appropriate introductions, take the time to sit down and talk with the patient. Establish an atmosphere of trust, using an optimistic but firm, realistic approach. Assess the patient's perception of what has and what will happen to him. Educate the patient about the role of therapy and what its function is. The patient needs to be reassured and given a full explanation of what is going to happen. Stress the importance of therapy: that we are not here to crush bones or as an instrument of torture, but rather to help him resume a normal life. Try to alleviate the patient's fear of moving his burned extremity because of the anticipation of pain, since fear can greatly jeopardize progress and hinder compliance. Stress the concept of independence and emphasize that successful rehabilitation is directly proportional to the patient's commitment to the rehabilitation process. It is now time for the therapist to finally perform the physical examination.

The basic premise in performing a physical examination is that the examiner, by use of all of his senses, can detect variations from the normal state. Physical examination should encompass the entire body. Each area should be inspected for probable areas of deformities and contractures prior to moving it.

Approach the uninvolved extremities first, in order to establish a baseline or norm for this particular patient. Assess the active range of motion. A goniometer may or may not be used, depending upon the location of the burn. Determining muscle strength is not appropriate, since it requires resistive exercise, which is generally contraindicated or impossible with acute burn patients.

Next, examine the head and neck. If dressing is present, gently remove it with the cooperation of the nursing staff. Observe for probable areas of deformities. For example, burns involving the sternocleidomastoid muscles or the anterior neck are guaranteed to produce severe limitations in neck extension and rotation (Fig. 2-4). Although there may be severe facial edema, it generally does not require special attention because of the natural elevated position of the bed.

Proceed to the anterior trunk area. Determine whether the configuration and location of the burn will impede lung expansion. Lung expansion may be reduced even if there is not a complete circumferential burn. Diaphragmatic breathing exercises are generally indicated to encourage lung expansion as well as stretching of the tissue over the thorax.

The shoulder and elbow should be examined next. The flexor surfaces of the shoulder and elbow, as well as the axilla, are the problematic areas, since inability to achieve full extension or neutral position occurs more readily than flexion limitations. Burns of the axilla or its anterior and posterior walls will also impede abduction (Fig. 2-5). Burns over the antecubital fossa predispose the patient towards flexion contractures (Fig. 2-6). Even if these joints are burned on the extensor surfaces, there should still be concern over extension limitation, since the patient will likely maintain a fetal position.

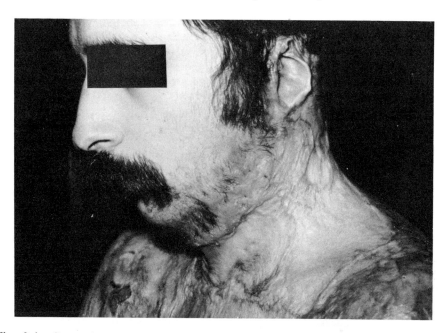

Fig. 2-4. Severe burn scar contractures of neck following third-degree burns and split-thickness skin graft to neck, chest, and shoulders.

Move on to the wrist and hand. During the examination, the hands should remain elevated to prevent edema. Observe the patient's hands to determine whether there are any exposed tendons, since ranging joints that are so damaged is prohibited. The attitude or resting position of the hand should be noted. This may reveal tendon damage. For example, if all of the digits except for one are flexed, flexor tendon damage should be suspected. Particular attention should be given to burns over the web spaces and palmar surface. The latter will possibly cause syndactyly or limitation of finger abduction, and the former could cause severe flexor contractures.

Following this inspection, evaluate the range of motion both actively and passively. Compare the contralateral findings for major discrepancies. Passive measurements can be expected to be greater than active measurements due to the patient's pain and fear of moving the fingers or a restricting edema.

Proceed to the lower extremities. Of particular concern are burns covering the inguinal fold, popliteal fossa, hamstrings, Achilles tendon, and the soles of the feet. Burns over the inguinal fold will encourage hip flexion; burns over the popliteal fossa or hamstrings will create knee flexion contractures; burns affecting the Achilles tendon will create heelcord contractures; and burns covering the soles of the feet will make ambulation prohibitive. Subsequent to inspection, measure active and passive range of motion. If ambulation has been cleared by the physician, use Ace wrap on both the involved and uninvolved lower extremities. Assess patient's transfer skills, including supine to sitting, sitting to standing, and vice versa, as well as bathroom transfer skills. Determine the type of assistance and devices that may be necessary

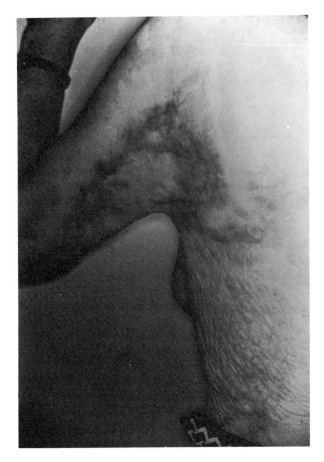

Fig. 2-5.   Burn scar contracture of axilla, limiting abduction of arm following burns and split-thickness skin graft to arm, axilla, and chest.

for ambulation. Check for gait deviations. Although crutches, canes, and walkers are not to be encouraged, they must certainly be considered.

The final information source to be approached is the patient's family. The family can give insight into the patient's psychosocial situation prior to the burn injury. Since patients adjust to the burn situation in a manner reflecting their total personality adjustment prior to injury,[6] this information should not be overlooked. By talking to the family, the patient's prior ability to adjust to stress and pain can be estimated. In addition, the question of whether the patient and his family are capable of coping with the burn and the resultant deformities can be considered.

Questions to ask the immediate family or next of kin should concern a history of alcohol and drug use, dominant figures in the patient's life, prior responses to stress and pain, and the patient's premorbid lifestyle. The answers to these questions will assist the staff in anticipating and coping with the patient's response to treatment.

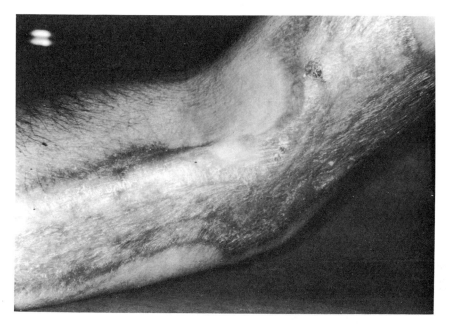

Fig. 2-6.   Burn scar contracture of elbow, limiting extension.

SELECTED MEDICAL PROCEDURES

Prior to the formulation of a therapy program, a discussion of certain medical procedures and standard physician orders is pertinent. The physician's basic initial orders concern fluid resuscitation and the maintainance of respiratory integrity, as well as care of the burn wound.

Fluid Resuscitation

The major pathophysiological attention following second- and third-degree burns is an increase in capillary permeability, resulting in loss of colloid, water, and electrolytes not only into the burn wound, but into unburned distant tissue as well.[4] Therefore, burn patients require enormous amounts of intravenous fluids in the immediate postburn period to restore intravascular volume and prevent hypovolemic shock. An intravenous line (I.V.) for fluid resuscitation and the placement of a Foley catheter to measure hourly urinary output are routinely included in the physician's admission orders for patients with greater than twenty percent total body surface area burns. The fluids are given intravenously, since oral replacement is impractical because of the volume of fluid required and that the majority of patients with major burns have a significant paralytic ileus during the first 48 to 72 hours postburn.[7] At a suitable time, the physician will place the I.V. in an area that will be least affected by immobilization. However, inasmuch as the I.V. should be placed in an unburned area to decrease the possibilities of infection, the physician may not have such a choice.

Since one of the signs of successful fluid resuscitation is adequate urine output, the orders will also include monitoring the patient's input and output. Usually the patient is not allowed oral supplementation for the first 24 hours or until there is positive evidence of active peristalsis and fluid balance has stabilized. When the patient is allowed oral fluids and nutrition, documentation of any intake during therapy should be made by the therapist or nursing staff on a flow sheet. In addition, the therapist should consult with the nursing staff prior to administering anything orally, since the patient may be requesting profuse amounts of fluids. Output will be monitored by the nursing staff, and therefore, the staff should be notified if and when the patient has voided.

Respiratory Integrity

Approximately 20 to 40 percent of burns treated at burn centers have some element of associated respiratory insult. Creating an artificial airway via an endotracheal tube or a tracheostomy is necessary when respiration must be supported by means of a ventilator. There are drawbacks to both approaches. The endotracheal tube is unstable in the active patient. Prolonged endotracheal intubation may lead to tracheomalacia and laryngeal stenosis, whereas a tracheostomy may lead to possible pneumonia from contamination by the burn wound, pneumothorax, massive atelectasis, or insensible water loss.[8,9] Despite the presence of a ventilator and endotracheal or tracheostomy tube, the physical therapy program must be initiated and continued.

Circulatory Integrity: Peripheral Vascular Considerations

A burned extremity is at risk not only from the burn of the overlying skin, but also from the adverse peripheral vascular circulatory consequences. Escharotomy, midlateral incisions of the constricting burn wound eschar, may be necessary to restore constricted circulation. Usually, involved extremities are elevated to reduce the production of dependent edema. Edema fluid appears to accumulate progressively during the first 24 to 36 hours postburn.[10–12] This edema formation is caused by direct vascular and lymphatic injury and is abetted by the accompanying increase in capillary permeability in nonburn tissues. In burns of less than 30 percent TBSA, the edema is generally confined to the burn area. However, burns involving greater than 30 percent TBSA produce edema that is distributed throughout all body tissues, with the amount being proportional to the magnitude of the injury. In both cases, the therapist must establish a position that provides optimal elevation, proper positioning, and exposure for treatments.

An escharotomy is an incision made through an eschar, usually in midlateral positions, to allow the underlying structures to expand. Since eschar does not possess normal elastic qualities, the development of relentless constricting edema caused by direct tissue injury, generalized increased capillary permeability, and large volumes of fluid resuscitation may be responsible for vascular compression. The physician

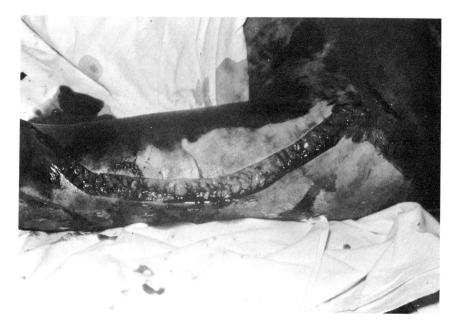

Fig. 2-7. Fresh escharotomy in circumferential burns of the upper extremity. Note how increased interstitial pressure of arm has forced apart the incision in the burned tissue.

will perform an escharotomy on patients with circumferential full-thickness burns of an extremity or chest wall. In the latter case, tissue edema will tighten the eschar until chest expansion and pulmonary ventilation expansion is restricted.

The extremity in question should be kept elevated and pulses checked hourly. If no pulse exists, an escharotomy should be performed. Since the tissue is nonviable, the procedure is generally painless and there is minimal bleeding. Following the procedure, the eschar will draw apart and permit expansion of the underlying compressed tissues and restoration of circulation (Fig. 2-7). Consequently, there will be improved color, temperature, sensation, motion, and peripheral pulses. The subsequent orders will include topical agents, elevation, and exercises.

Cleansing Techniques

Tanking, showering, and sponge bathing are common techniques used to cleanse the burn wound. Tanking refers to the total immersion of the patient in a whirlpool or Hubbard tank. Showering refers to high-pressure irrigation of the patient from a hand-held shower head. Sponge bathing is performed bedside and is self-explanatory. The common goal of all three techniques is to keep the wound clean, remove dead tissue, bacteria, and caked antimicrobials. One of the three cleansing techniques is usually performed every shift.

The ability to remove bacteria from infected wounds is one of the primary benefits of hydrotherapy, specifically tanking.[13] Additional benefits of hydrotherapy include:

1. Relatively painless dressing removal,
2. Accurate assessment of TBSA and depth of burn,
3. Softening and debriding eschar,
4. Relaxation and pain reduction,
5. Assisting with extremity exercise,
6. Use as a transmission agent for electrolytes and other chemicals,[14]
7. Favorably influencing metabolic functions,[14]
8. Total body cleansing

These benefits can only be realized if the treatment is performed properly with appropriate concern for safety and maintenance of body heat, and if the patient can tolerate this activity. Tanking is obviously not indicated for patients with tracheostomies or endotracheal tubes.

Tanking may be performed by the therapist or the nursing staff, contingent upon the policy of the particular institution. The Hubbard tank should be in an isolated treatment room that is maintained at 29°C with heat lamps. During the entire treatment procedure, sterile technique is strictly adhered to. For this reason, whirlpools are not used, as it is extremely difficult to keep the agitators free of bacteria, especially water borne *Praudonoras* sp.

At the Burn Center at Nassau County Medical Center, the tank is prepared by covering it with a disposable plastic liner that has two airways incorporated into its design. These airways allow for customized agitation by enabling the therapist or nurse to create holes for air agitation at the desired location. Tubes from an air compressor are placed in each of the two pathways. The water stretcher (plinthe) is also encased in a disposable liner and placed on top of a wheel stretcher. The single-use disposable liners protect against cross-contamination. The tank is filled halfway with 95 to 100°F tap water, depending on the patient's tolerance. This temperature range is acceptable because it gives the patient a neutral to warm sensation.[15]

At this time, the hydrotherapy room is ready to receive the patient. The patient is transferred to the hydrotherapy room via the prepared stretcher. The dressing gown and outer layer of dressings are removed and the remaining dressings are gently slit. The patient is transferred to and from the tank by an overhead electric hoist and a specially prepared plinthe. Once the patient is in the tank, the compressor is turned on and the remaining dressings removed (Fig. 2-8).

Removing the dressings while the patient is immersed produces minimal discomfort, thereby decreasing metabolic demands.[14] Following dressing removal, the wound should be inspected for areas of change that suggest wound degeneration or bacterial invasion. Following this inspection and depending on the patient's tolerance, gentle active and active assistive range of motion exercises should be performed for a maximum of ten minutes. A maximum time is specified because the patient should not be submerged for longer than 25 minutes. Prolonged periods of tanking with tap water can result in a considerable metabolic imbalance from the transfer of sodium, phosphorus, and calcium ions between the wound surface and the water.[14] Some patients find the tank to be relaxing and soothing, whereas others associate it with debridement and pain.

Directly after exercising or wound inspection, the patient is cleansed and, if

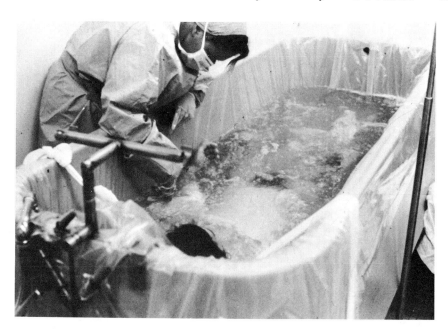

Fig. 2-8. Patient being treated in hydrotherapy tank. Hydrotherapy tanks are useful for cleansing, debriding and evaluating burns. In addition, this form of therapy often increases the patient's sense of well-being.

indicated, the burn wound is debrided to the point of pain and bleeding. The patient is then lifted by the electric hoist to just above the surface of the water. Loose debris is removed by gentle irrigation with a standard whirlpool rinse-out hose. An investigation by Niederhuber and associates suggests that this method is of value in removing bacteria, nonviable tissue fragments, and foreign matters from wounds.[16] The patient is then transferred to a stretcher draped with a sterile sheet. The wound is allowed to air dry or is blotted dry with a sterile towel. Heat lamps may be necessary after tanking, since the loss of heat due to surface evaporation may drop the patient's temperature to 94°F or below.[17] The prescribed topical agent may then be applied, dressings reapplied, and the patient returned to his room.

When tanking is not indicated, showering may be the treatment of choice. Its primary benefits are similar to those of tanking in that it aids in dressing removal, cleansing, burn wound assessment, exercising, and debridement. However, patients rarely find the treatment relaxing or their pain reduced.

Every patient room in our Burn Center has a showering room. The patient is asked to ambulate or propel himself to the shower room using a wheelchair. If the patient is on bedrest because of lower extremity burns, showering is still performed, using a wheelchair with elevated leg rests. The patient is transferred to a tub chair, keeping the lower extremities elevated on a second tub chair, and the dressing gown and outer dressings are removed. The patient is lavaged with a hand-held shower spray, and the remaining dressings removed. This is succeeded by spot debridement and cleansing. The spray is turned off, the patient is dried with sterile towels, and the appropriate dressings are reapplied. Exercises can be performed in the shower room prior to dressing application or after the patient returns to bed.

Sponge bathing bedside is reserved for those patients who are unresponsive, on respirators, immobilized by recent grafting procedures, or on absolute bedrest.

Dressings

Depending upon the policy of the burn center, light dressings, bulky dressings, or no dressings may be used. If dressings are not employed, then physical therapy sessions may be scheduled at any time convenient to the therapist or patient. However, if light or bulky dressings are used, then it is best to coordinate therapy sessions with the nursing staff. The preferred time for physical therapy sessions are usually immediately after dressing removal and hydrotherapy sessions. Debridement is usually performed at this time also; however, it is probably best to do physical therapy routines before debridement because of the pain that is sometimes associated with debridement.

Debridement Techniques

Sepsis is the most common cause of late morbidity and mortality in the burn patient. In order to prevent this complication, debridement is performed routinely. Its purpose is to minimize sepsis by hastening the removal of nonviable tissue at the interface of the living and dead tissue, and to ready the wound for ultimate coverage. Debridement can be accomplished mechanically, surgically, or by topical chemical enzymes, while in the operating room, at the bedside, or during hydrotherapy sessions.

The most conservative and effective method of debridement is mechanical debridement. This is usually done with scalpels, scissors, and forceps by the medical staff, nursing staff, or the therapist during hydrotherapy sessions. The water and scrubbing helps to loosen and soften the eschar. Forceps are used to lift the loosened eschar, while scalpel or scissors excise it at the viable-nonviable interface. All necrotic loose tissue is trimmed away, stopping at the point of bleeding or pain. In most cases, there is minimal blood loss; however, occasionally bleeding persists. In these cases, pressure is applied by hand or dressings, with the latter being checked frequently for continued blood loss.

Another method of mechanical debridement is wet to dry saline dressings. This method is commonly used as a final preparation of the burn wound prior to grafting. With this technique, dressings soaked in saline solution are placed on the wound, allowed to dry, and then removed. As the dry dressings are removed, small pieces of necrotic tissue that have adhered to the dressings are also removed. It is most effective when all eschar has been removed except for small fragments of necrotic debris on the wound surface. If there is a significant delay before going to the operating room for grafting, antimicrobials must be resumed or pigskin applied to the wound to prevent infection. When exercise is indicated, it should be performed when the dressings have been removed or soon after dressing changes, when the dressings are still wet and supple.

A more aggressive method of debridement is formal surgical debridement performed in the operating room. Surgical debridement has become an increasingly utilized method of wound management in patients with deep dermal injury.[18] Its purpose is to decrease the patient's liability to invasive burn wound sepsis by attempting burn wound closure in the shortest period of time prior to invasion of the burn wound by bacteria.

There are two types of surgical debridement, tangential excision and primary excision, both of which are performed under general or regional anesthesia. *Tangential excision* refers to a technique in which the necrotic tissue of a deep partial-thickness burn is removed in sequential layers to a base of viable dermis. Split-thickness skin grafts may then be applied immediately or delayed for 24 hours. In *primary excision,* the surgeon removes necrotic tissue down to the level of deep fascia. It should be performed before the fifth day postburn, since bacteria colonization is at a minimum prior to that time and bleeding is less.

In either case, after debridement the wounds are covered for 24 hours with either pigskin or saline soaks. This helps to control bleeding and insures homeostasis at the subsequent grafting sessions. Twenty-four to forty-eight hours later, the patient is brought back to the operating room for the placement of split-thickness autografts.

When successful, surgical debridement decreases the length of hospitalization, helps prevent scar contractures, allows for early motion, and minimizes the likelihood of burn wound sepsis. However, there are several drawbacks. With tangential excision, there may be massive blood loss, difficulty in determining the exact depth of burn, and the risk of multiple general anesthesias. Some of the disadvantages of primary excision are significant bleeding, lack of donor sites, risk of general anesthesia, and the creation of new donor sites, which are a potential source of infection.

A more recently developed method of debridement is enzymatic debridement. This entails the use of a proteolytic enzymatic debriding agent that proponents claim will rapidly digest necrotic tissue without harming adjacent healthy tissue. Conclusive evidence of the value of enzymatic debridement as a consistently useful tool has yet to be supplied.

The most common enzyme used for ezymatic debridement is sutilains ointment (Travase). When using enzymes, they are applied from the day of admission to approximately the sixth day. In our Burn Center, enzymes are used in the following fashion. The patient is cleansed without betadine scrubs (heavy-metal agents are contraindicated) and dried with sterile towels. A thick layer of enzyme is applied with sterile gloves. If an antimicrobial is indicated, mesh gauze impregnated with silver sulfadiazine is applied over the enzyme. This is wrapped with Kerlix gauze followed by Kling gauze. While Travase is being used to soften the eschar prior to primary excision, the enzyme is covered with saline-soaked towels for 24 hours, with dressing changes every 8 hours. In both cases, it is extremely important to keep the enzyme moist, since it functions more effectively in that fashion.

The greatest advantage of Travase is its effectiveness in the treatment of deep partial-thickness dorsal hand burns. It is applied immediately postburn and covered with plastic wrap. After 24 hours, the eschar is soft and ready to be scraped off, rather than cut off in the operating room. Immediately following debridement and cleansing, the hand is ready to receive the split-thickness grafts.[19]

Theoretically, enzymes seem to be the ideal way to remove eschar in that they require neither an anesthetic nor a surgical procedure. However, there are many disadvantages. There is an increase in fluid loss when Travase is applied early after the thermal injury.[19] Consequently, the patient must be monitored judiciously. Enzymes can only be used over limited surface areas. They induce blood loss from the small thrombosed capillaries that are reopened. Most importantly, after enzyme treatment, the wound bed may not be suitable to accept a skin graft. The enzyme merely debrides down to the subcutaneous fat. Skin grafting cannot be done without first excising the remaining devitalized tissue or allowing time for spontaneous sloughing and the development of adequate granulation tissue.[19]

Whether mechanical, surgical, or enzymatic debridement is employed depends on the medical status of the patient and the individual characteristics of the burn wound. The goal of the three methods remains the same: the removal of nonviable tissue as quickly as possible without jeopardizing the status of the patient. Once this goal is met, the patient will be ready to receive the skin grafts with resulting burn wound coverage.

Grafting

Once a satisfactory recipient area has been prepared either by mechanical, surgical, or enzymatic debridement or tissue slough, the wound is ready for skin grafting. Frequently, burn wound biopsies will be performed to ensure that tissue bacterial levels at the recipient site are sufficiently low to allow "take" of the valuable grafts.

Split-thickness skin grafts are usually performed in the operating room. The grafts are taken with a hand-powered or mechanically powered device called a *dermatome*. This device harvests split thickness of skin between 10 and 25 thousandths of an inch from an unburned area called a *donor site*. The donor sites are then usually covered with some form of dressing or left exposed. Donor sites may be considered to be an additional area of partial-thickness skin loss and may represent another source of difficulty for the therapist, as they are a source of pain and frequently limit motion at that point. Nevertheless, the site must be treated with great care, since the ultimate survival of a patient with a significant burn depends upon the rapid and frequent reharvesting of skin from the same donor location.

The harvested split-thickness skin grafts are then applied in the operating room with sutures, staples, or mesh,[20] and are usually covered with a dressing (Fig. 2-9).[20] The grafted part may or may not be splinted or immobilized. Depending upon the location and burn facility policy, physical therapy programs to that area may commence three to five days after grafting. It must be remembered that these areas are still vulnerable to damage at this time, and great care should be observed when dealing with recently grafted areas.

DEVELOPING A TREATMENT PROGRAM

Although preserving optimal function and range of motion throughout burn treatment is a universal goal, specific goals are unique to each patient. Some patients may be ambulatory during the postgraft stage, and others may be confined to bed or in traction (Fig. 2-10). Therefore, an individualized treatment program must be developed and carried out to effectively and efficiently achieve the specified goals.

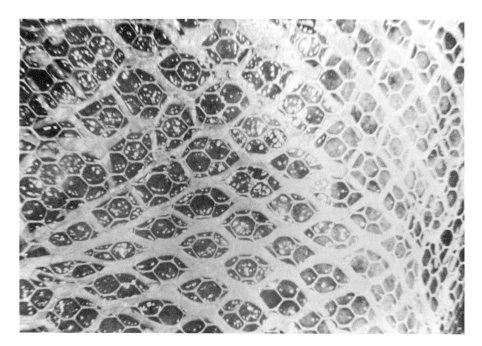

Fig. 2-9. Meshed split-thickness skin graft being treated with meshed nylon overdressing to minimize shear force to grafts during dressing changes.

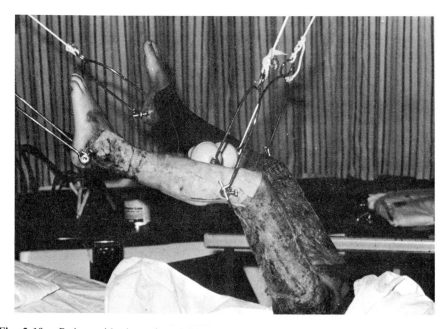

Fig. 2-10. Patient with circumferential burns of lower extremities in overhead traction after skin grafting. Such an apparatus minimizes shear forces on grafts and allows for ease of dressing changes and inspection of wounds.

The treatment program should take into account all of the data compiled during the evaluation process. In addition, the therapist must consider the constraints and limitations of time, number of staff members, and other impediments to the attainment of the desired goals. This section will discuss the development of a treatment program, emphasizing the goals of minimizing joint deformities and maximizing the patient's functional independence.

Minimizing Joint Deformities

Joint range of motion and proper positioning of the patient in bed are of paramount importance if joint deformities are to be prevented. A judicious balance between positioning the patient to maintain the end of the range most susceptible to contracture formation and movement to maintain the other end of range will produce the most desirable results.[21]

The purpose of splinting and positioning is to reinforce functional positions and prevent the accomodation of soft tissue structures to shortened positions. The program should continue until the wound is closed and the patient can attain the complete range of motion and maintain it for a period of time without a splint.

Points to consider when positioning include:

1. *Depth and Location of Burn.* This information will assist in anticipating the direction of the deformities. Partial-thickness and full-thickness burns exhibit different properties in the acute patient. Initially, partial-thickness burns are elastic and pliable, whereas full-thickness burns are nonelastic and thicker. The location of the burn is the major determinant of positioning. Of important concern are those patients with burns that cross the flexor surface of the joint, or burns lateral to this surface. These burns will display stronger deformity tendencies than burns of the extensor surface.

2. *Location and Degree of Edema.* This information will determine the extent of elevation required.

3. *Desired Position of Extremities.* This position will be different for each patient. The cardinal rule is that the position of comfort is inevitably the position that most encourages contracture. Characteristically, the burn patient attempts to maintain a fetal position, one of flexion and adduction. Subsequently, those patients with burns that cross the flexor or lateral surface are of greatest concern.

4. *Desired Trunk Position.* This position will be determined by the optimal position of the extremities, cardiopulmonary status, potential decubiti sites, and the location of any trunk burns. Modifications will have to be made for respiratory or cardiac problems, respirators, I.V.'s, and so on. A poor cardiopulmonary status will require maintaining the patient in a semivertical position. Elderly patients with thin skin are ideally kept off their sacrum or on a support system. Patients with posterior trunk burns will be more comfortable lying on their side or prone.

5. *Methods Available.* Decisions regarding what methods are going to best achieve the desired position must be made. Splinting, towels, pillows, foam pads, I.V. suspension sling, and bedside tables are some of the options that are available.

6. *Positioning Schedule.* The patient's mental status, motivation, activity level,

and tolerance will determine how long and at what times the splints must be worn. Even if the patient is capable of exercising independently, positioning and splinting should still be carried out during periods of rest and sleep. This will discourage soft tissue accomodation to the patient's position of comfort.

The following case study is an example of a positioning program initiated in our unit. A 25-year-old male was admitted to the Burn Center at Nassau County Medical Center with partial- and full-thickness burns incurred 4 hours ago. Both hands had partial-thickness burns over the dorsum, extending to the DIP's. The right upper extremity had circumferential deep dermal burns up to, but not including, the axilla. The left upper extremity had deep dermal burns extending posteriorly two inches proximal to the olecranon. Both lower extremities and trunk were spared. The patient also suffered partial-thickness burns to the neck and face. He had no significant previous medical history; however, it was assumed that there was an inhalation component because of the presence of facial burns.

The patient was positioned as follows. Both hands were placed in interim prefabricated cockup splints and elevated with I.V. poles and pillows to deter extensive edema formation. Even though the burns were on the posterior aspect of the left elbow, care was taken to position both elbows with as much extension as possible. The inhalation component necessitated a semivertical position. Accomodation for the neck burns included a very narrow rolled towel under the neck to encourage hyperextension. The patient was instructed to raise his trunk off the bed hourly to prevent decubiti, as well as to insure proper active positioning of his lower extremities. The patient was placed in a reverse Trendelenburg periodically for postural drainage. The I.V. poles were discontinued seven days post admission when edema had subsided.

Subsequent to the formation of a position program, plans for exercise implementation must be devised to further minimize the possibility of joint deformities. What? when? where? and how? must be determined. The answers are dependent upon the medical condition of the patient. Keep in mind that the primary modality of the therapist is exercise to maintain function and decrease edema.

Points to consider when exercising include:

1. *What Joints Must Be Exercised and in What Planes.* This will be determined by the location and configuration of the burn. Joint integrity will be maintained by exercising individual joints with the underlying tissues and musculature in a relaxed position. Maximum stretching of the tissues and musculature can be achieved by performing multiaxial exercises.

2. *What Type of Exercise Is Indicated.* In order of preference, the choices are active, active assistive, and passive range of motion. Active exercise is most desirable because it can meet the needs of the patient and incite the minimal amount of stress. Active assistive exercise is necessary for patients who are unable to achieve full range of motion actively, or who cannot tolerate the demands of an active exercise program. Passive range of motion exercise is reserved for comatose patients or extremely uncooperative patients; it is rarely indicated in deep partial- or full-thickness burns to the hands unless specifically ordered. Resistive exercise is usually not indicated until the patient is out of the acute stage.

3. *Where the Exercises Should Be Performed.* If the patient is confined to bed because of a respirator, lower extremity burns, or grafting, exercising must be performed in bed. If not, there are several options. Exercising during tanking or showering is advantageous in that the patient is not restricted by cumbersome bandages. Additional alternatives are exercising while sitting or standing in the patient's room or adjoining facilities. Keep in mind the problem of edema formation when making this decision—elevation must be maintained as consistently as possible.

4. *When Exercises Should Be Performed.* This depends on the nursing schedule of the patient and what time of day the patient is most tolerant of exercise. Discussion with the nursing staff as well as the patient will provide the answer. If the exercises are to be performed during tanking or showering, or immediately following the dressing change, ask the staff to accommodate themselves to the therapy schedule.

5. *Duration and Frequency of Exercise.* This depends on the patient's tolerance, motivation, and nursing schedule. It is easier to prevent tightness and maintain range of motion by frequently repeated activity than to correct it after it has developed. Ideally, the patient should receive no less than two structured exercise sessions a day, seven days a week.

Maximizing Independence

Successful performance of ambulation and self-care tasks by the burn patient provides a strong incentive to seek further independence. Both increase the patient's sense of well-being, stimulate appetite, assist in pulmonary toileting, ease dependency on the nursing staff, as well as augmenting range of motion exercises. Physiologically,

> the biochemical changes in metabolism caused by trauma are compounded by inactivity. Inactivity causes alterations in the fluid compartments, in electrolyte balance and in circulation. It contributes to an increased nitrogen loss and muscular wasting, to a change in mineral content of bone and a decrease in resting metabolic expenditure. The decrease in energy requirements associated with inactivity is rarely adequate to counteract the increased energy requirements caused by trauma.[22]

Throughout the entire course of the patient's recovery from a burn injury, self-care should be encouraged and reinforced by all professionals involved. Self-care assists the patient in reaching the common goal of achieving maximum function. In addition, family education and cooperation is necessary so that the family will not interfere by doing everything for the patient in a misguided sense of compassion. Such interference will undermine the staff's approach, as well as be detrimental to the patient.

Activities that the patient can do independently, such as eating and assisting in dressing changes, should be required as soon as realistically possible. If the patient has suffered lower extremity burns, he may be confined to bed during the rescusitation stage because of obligatory edema. In these cases, self-care tasks while in bed are emphasized.

Independent transfers and ambulation should be initiated as soon as medically permissable. This will aid in maintaining range of motion, prevent disuse atrophy of the lower extremities, promote circulation, and decrease the patient's sense of dependency. Each patient must be evaluated to determine whether his tolerance and medical condition will permit this type of demanding activity. Points to consider when considering ambulation include:

1. *Cardiopulmonary Status.* Will ambulation put too much demand on the heart and lungs? Obviously, this decision demands consultation with the burn team in its entirety.

2. *Extent of Edema.* If there is severe edema in the lower extremities, ambulation might be delayed. Ace wraps are indicated in all lower extremity burns, whatever the extent of edema. This will also help prevent venous stasis.

3. *I.V. Lines, Respirators, etc.* Such items will necessitate extra help with ambulation or prevent ambulation.

4. *Cooperation and Pain Tolerance.* Ambulation requires a certain level of cooperation from the patient to make it an acceptable modality. If the patient's pain tolerance is minimal, ambulation may create an undue amount of stress, which would make it an undesirable initial activity. Any effort to force the patient to ambulate is detrimental to his mental well-being and the patient-therapist rapport.

5. *Assistive Devices.* Although crutches, canes, and walkers are not encouraged, certain patients may require their assistance.

Resumption of self-care activities and ambulation as soon as tolerable is vital in preventing general debilitation and the secondary complications of prolonged bedrest. Their greatest benefit, however, lies in the emotional uplift and sense of well-being they provide.

RATIONALE FOR EARLY INTERVENTION

The key to rehabilitative success of the severely burned patient is the *early* introduction of both physical and occupational therapy. Although physical therapy is an ongoing process, it is imperative that aggressive physical therapy through positioning and exercise be started immediately. An early intensive exercise program under a physical therapist's supervision can give the patient the best chance of surviving his injury with minimal loss of function.[21]

Starting the exercise program immediately after admission offers many advantages. First, there is a better chance of preventing overwhelming deformities and contractures. It has been documented that one of the primary factors that influences morbidity is the length of time elapsing before postburn physical therapy is initiated.[21] Second, the effects of immobilization and edema can be greatly reduced when vigorous active range of motion is initiated within the first 24 to 48 hours.[11,21,23] This is because edema fluid appears to accumulate progressively during the first 24 to 36 hours postburn; and if allowed to persist, fibrosis of muscle and joint structures will occur.[11,17,21] Frequent and early introduction of active range of motion exercises will help to rid the area of edema by increasing its venous return.[12] Third, working toward preventing joint restrictions and resulting deformities is less arduous a task than dealing with them after they occur.

Further considerations for initiating physical therapy are the psychological benefits that can be gained. Early motion will counter the patient's initial concept that their burned extremity cannot be moved.[24] Initiating and explaining proper positioning early in burn care will help the patient to accept these positions as desirable, and give him a feeling that he is participating in his own recovery.

REFERENCES

1. Perry RR, Buffler PA, Sanderson LM: A research model for the study of rehabilitation among adult burn injury patients. Rehab Lit 43:77–80, 1982
2. Dobbs ER, Curreri WP: Burns, analysis of results of physical therapy in 681 patients. J Trauma 12:242–248, 1972
3. Tobiasen J, Hiebert J, O'Brien R, Edlich R: A graded risk index of burn severity. J Burn Care 1:31–35, 1980
4. Munster AM: Burn Care for the House Officer. Baltimore, Williams & Wilkens, 1980
5. Miller WC, Gardner N, Mlott SR: Psychosocial support in the treatment of severely burned patients. J Trauma 16:722–25, 1976
6. Lewis SR, Goolishian HA, Wolf CW, Lynch JB, Blocker TG: Psychological studies in burn patients. Plast & Reconstruct Surg 31:323, 1963
7. Yarbrough DR: Pathophysiology of the burn wound. p 29. In: Care of the Burn-Injured Patient, ed. Wagner MM. Littleton, PSG Publishing Co., 1981
8. Tanigawa MC, et al: The burned hand: a physical therapy protocol. Phys Ther 54(9):953–958, 1974
9. Gronley, J: Early intensive physical therapy for the burned hand. Phys Ther 44(10):875–880, 1964
10. Krizek TJ: Care of the burned patient. pp584–643. In: The Management of Trauma, eds. Ballinger WF, Rutherford RB, Zuidema GD. Philadelphia, WB Saunders, 1968
11. Salisbury RE, Dingeldein GP: Early management of the burned upper extremity. Current Concepts in Trauma Care 3(1):16–21, 1980
12. Salisbury RE, Loveless S., Silverstein P., Wilmore DW, Moylan JA, Pruitt BA: Postburn edema of the upper extremity: evaluation of present treatment. J Trauma 13:857–862, 1973
13. Bohannon RW: Whirlpool versus whirlpool and rinse for removal of bacteria from a stasis ulcer. Phys Ther 62(3):304–308, 1982
14. Headley BJ, Robson MC, Krizek TJ: Methods of reducing environmental stress for the acute burn patient. Phys Ther 55(1):5–9, 1975
15. Behrend HJ: Hydrotherapy. pp239–253. In: Medical Hydrology, ed. Licht S. Baltimore, Waverly Press, 1963
16. Niederhuber SS, Stribley RF, Koepke GH: Reduction of skin bacterial load with use of therapeutic whirlpool. Phys Ther 55:482–486, 1975
17. Roberts ML, Pruitt BA: Nursing care & psychological considerations. p 378. In: Burns A Team Approach, eds. Artz CP, Moncrief JA, Pruitt BA. Philadelphia, WB Saunders, 1979

18. Baxter CR: Early surgical excision and immediate grafting. p 224. In: Burns A Team Approach, eds. Artz CP, Moncrief JA, Pruitt BA. Philadelphia, W.B. Saunders Co., 1979
19. Gant TD: The early enzymatic debridement and grafting of deep dermal burns to the hand. Presented at the Annual Meeting of Amer. Soc. of Plastic and Reconstruct Surgeons. Toronto, Oct. 10, 1979
20. DiGregorio VR: Meshed nylon overdressings for sutureless skin grafting. Annals of Plastic Surgery 1(4): p 429–430, July, 1978
21. Jaeger DL: Maintenance of function of the burn patient. Phys Ther 52:627–633, 1972
22. Long CL, Bonilla LE: Metabolic effects of inactivity and injury. p 209. In: Physiology of Rehabilitation, eds. Downey J, Darling R. Philadelphia, WB Saunders, 1971
23. Hoopes JE: The recovery from burns. pp 643–658. In: The Management of Trauma, eds. Ballinger WF, Rutherford RB, Zuidema GD. Philadelphia, WB Saunders, 1968
24. Helm PA, et al: Burn rehabilitation—a team approach. Surg Clin NA 58(6):1236–1277, 1978

3 | Occupational Therapy: Splinting, Positioning, and Exercise

Nora Goldberg
Patti Stadler
Mitch Kaplan

A discussion of burn injury requires a broad understanding of the scope of the problem. Although it is difficult to obtain accurate statistics, current literature estimates that there are approximately two million burn incidents (injury, death, disability) per year, half of which require prolonged hospitalization.[1] The need for specialized hospital care has led to the establishment of burn treatment centers, where significant advances in medical management and specially trained burn teams have improved the survival rates of patients with extensive burns. Whether a burn victim returns to a normal productive existence depends upon both the extent and depth of the burn injury and the patient's management by the burn team.

The burn team consists of all of the health care professionals involved in the patient's care. In the contained burn unit, this team is usually composed of a surgeon, nurse, physical therapist, occupational therapist, dietition, psychiatrist, and social worker. The overall objective of the burn team is to preserve life and minimize morbidity. The specific objective of the therapist, as a member of the team, is to preserve function and provide emotional support throughout and beyond hospitalization. In this chapter, we will discuss the role of the therapist, the specific goals of treatment throughout the different phases of healing, and the treatment program. Exercise and splinting of specific joints will be organized anatomically (upper extremity burns, lower extremity burns, and special areas—head, neck, and face burns), taking the reader chronologically through the stages of healing.

THE ROLE OF OCCUPATIONAL THERAPY

Maintaining Physical Function

The primary goal of therapy is early and complete restoration of physical function. This is accomplished by exercise, directed activities, and proper positioning of joints during periods of rest or immobilization. Additional responsibilities include understanding and assisting the burn team with wound care, specifically cleaning, debriding, and dressing the burns during the acute phase and instructing the patient in skin precautions after grafting.

Providing Psychological Support

The secondary goal, of all members of the burn team, is to help the patient effectively deal with the emotional consequences of the burn injury and its treatment. Understanding the patient's feelings and helping him to develop adequate coping mechanisms increases compliance with the therapy program.

The burn injury is an unexpected and catastrophic event for the patient and his family. The situation is frequently complicated by feelings of guilt for the carelessness or ignorance that may have caused the accident. As in all illnesses, patients express feelings of anxiety and depression, and may at times display aggressive behavior.[2] There is fear of additional suffering from the treatments (hydrotherapy, dressing changes, and therapy sessions). Thus, those individuals who represent the forces of healing also represent the instruments of torture to the patient. There are feelings of depression related to loss of self-image, separation from family, loss of income, and potential permanent disfigurement. This stressed emotional state may make it difficult for the patient to comprehend and participate in the therapy program.

To obtain maximal patient cooperation and set the tone for future sessions, the therapist must gain the patient's trust during early interactions. During the initial treatment session, the therapist should explain the nature and extent of the injury, the anticipated healing process, the rationale for therapy, and the need for clearly defined goals. It is important to address the patient's concerns regarding painful treatment and be supportive and explain procedures, but not allow sympathy to limit the goals of treatment. When the critical phase is over, the patient should be encouraged to assume as much responsibility as is possible for independence and self-care. This may include having the patient assist with wound care or dressing changes, and having the patient perform independent ranging exercises in addition to the formal therapy sessions.

With prolonged hospitalization, the therapist's continued support is needed to maintain the patient's motivation. This is especially important during periods of isolation, medical set back, immobilization, and pain. It is important to remember that in burn therapy complications delaying recovery are the rule rather than the exception.

Anticipated hospital discharge begins a new, difficult, stressful situation. During the crisis period of confinement in the burn center, the patient has developed close and frequently dependent relationships with members of the burn team. The focus has been on healing and maintaining function. With the prospect of returning home, the patient begins to realize the effect that his disability and disfigurement will have on future functioning and interpersonal relationships. The continued posthospitalization therapeutic relationship with the therapist serves to encourage independence and increased self-esteem while maximizing physical functioning.

THE THERAPY PROGRAM

The goal of the therapy program is to maintain physical function throughout healing. The therapist must anticipate potential impairment and provide early treatment (exercise and splinting) to prevent functional and cosmetic deformity. Deformity may occur from skin and soft tissue contracture, destruction of tendon and muscle, orthopedic complications, and changes related to prolonged immobilization. Treatment should begin on the first day of admission with structured therapy sessions for 20 to 30 minutes twice a day.

Contractures

The normal healing process involves contracture and scarring. During this process, fibroblasts and myofibroblasts proliferate and move toward the cell-free center of the wound. Healing proceeds with contracture of the injured area, leading to ultimate reduction in wound size. The opposing forces of vigorous active exercise and splinting are needed to counteract the contracting forces.

As the scar tissue matures, fibroblasts lay down inelastic collagen tissue, causing further contracture and hypertrophic scarring. This phase peaks from three to six months postburn and continues until full maturation of the scar has occurred.

Prevention of Deformity

Throughout the healing process of the burn, frequent exercise, splinting, and compression (in the later stage) are needed to preserve tissue length, range of motion, and therefore, function.

Exercise

Patients are instructed and assisted in exercises that put the involved joint (the term *involved joint* refers to a joint affected because of injury to the skin covering it) and adjacent joints through complete range of motion. Early active range of motion exercises are preferred. If a patient's fear of pain limits his ability to perform active exercises, then the therapist may assist active movement to obtain full range of motion (active assistive exercise). Muscle strengthening exercises may be indicated to prevent disuse atrophy. Resistive exercise, mat activities, and modified proprioceptive neuromuscular facilitation (PNF) techniques have been useful methods to maintain range of motion.[1] Passive range of motion (the therapist moves the joint without patient assistance) is used as a last resort in the unresponsive patient. Vigorous passive ranging is contraindicated. Forceful movements can rupture fine muscle fibers and vessels surrounding the joint, producing a hematoma within the joint space that may lead to fibrosis or heterotopic calcification.

Activities

While exercise programs focus on maintaining joint range of motion and muscle tone, functional activity may be needed to preserve the normal pattern of movement and guard against compensated motion due to pain. Adapted crafts and games can be used to encourage hand function. They can provide an interesting way to increase the amount of time spent using the involved part, increase self-esteem, involve family members in treatment, and offer an alternative to constant focus on the burn. The type of activity may have to be modified for sterile considerations and is always dependent on the patient's interest and ability to concentrate.

Edema Control

All significant burns involve edema of varying degrees. Protein-rich edema fluid penetrates elastic tissue, tendon sheaths, fascial coverings, and joint capsules and becomes trapped in fibrous tissue. Prolonged edema ultimately leads to fibrosis and restricted movement. Elevation and early active movement will reduce edema. Severe edema, in which circulation is compromised, may require surgical escharotomy. This should be followed by elevation of the extremity and a vigorous exercise regimen.

Edema control is easily accomplished during night and bedrest by elevation positioning (Fig. 3-1). During the day, the ambulatory patient must understand the importance of elevation and assume this responsibility. A noncompliant patient may require an axilla splint for daytime elevation (see section on axilla burns).

Activities of Daily Living

The contractile forces involved in wound closure are relentless. In addition to structured exercise, the patient must be encouraged to actively use the involved part throughout the day. This requires the coordinated effort of the entire team. Assistive devices may be fabricated by the occupational therapist to enable the patient with limited movement to gain independence and self-care.

SPLINTING

As an adjunct to the therapy program or during periods of enforced immobilization, splints are used to provide support and proper position and to maintain ideal skin and ligament length. The need for a splint is initially determined by depth of the burn and joint involvement and must be constantly reevaluated throughout the course of treatment. Contracture deformities can be prevented by early splinting.

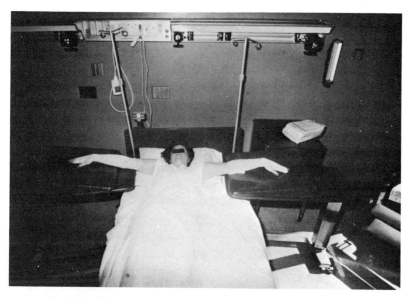

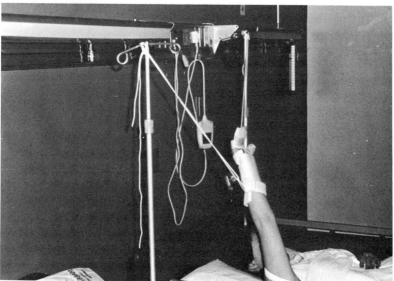

Fig. 3-1. Positioning for edema control in the upper extremity.

Materials

Splints may be fabricated out of commercially available low temperature thermoplastic materials. In the early stages of the burn, when the contour of the extremity changes frequently, easily remolded splints will make the task of the therapist easier.

Application

Splints should be applied over dressings and secured with gauze or Ace wrap. All nursing shifts must be instructed in their proper application. The splints must be checked frequently for pressure spots and circulatory impairment. Absorbent padding should be avoided, as the splints then become wet and retain bacteria. The splints must be thoroughly cleaned at each dressing change to minimize bacterial risk.

Types of Splints

Primary Splints. During the acute phase and pregrafting period, static splints (without movable parts) are used to position the involved joints during sleep, inactivity, or periods of unresponsiveness. Whenever possible, these splints should be applied to adjacent intact skin and those surfaces with the least amount of injury. Primary splinting should be simple so that fabrication can be accomplished quickly, and application can be managed efficiently by the nursing staff during this busy period. It is best to avoid fabrication directly on the patient. Generally accepted principles can be followed for positioning extremities in splints during the acute stage.[3] The position may need to be altered depending upon the nature and location of the burns in each individual patient.

During the critical stage, splints are worn continuously until the patient is able to perform frequent self-mobilization exercise. As the patient assumes increased responsibility for exercise and independent self-care, splints are removed during the day and worn only at rest and sleep. If full range of motion is not maintained, continuous wearing of splints may be needed.

Postgraft Splints. During the immediate postgraft phase, splints are used to immobilize joints in proper position, but must allow access for continued wound care. The need for the splint must be anticipated. The splint is fabricated prior to surgery in accordance with the anticipated surgical plan and applied in the operating room immediately after grafting. These splints are worn continuously for five to fourteen days until the graft is secure.

Follow-Up Splints. The chronic phase of burn care begins with wound closure and continues until full maturation of the wound (one to two years). Static splinting may be continued during this period to insure full range of motion. If the patient is maintained on a therapy program and does not show loss of movement, splinting may be decreased to night periods only and ultimately discontinued.

Dynamic splints (movable parts) are used to increase function. They can provide support to the joint without restricting antagonistic movements, provide slow steady force to stretch a skin contracture, or provide resistive force for exercise.

SPLINTING AND EXERCISE FOR THE UPPER EXTREMITY

Axilla

Early Considerations.   Burns in the axilla or adjacent tissue areas are well-known for developing contractures that limit arm function.[4] During the acute phase, the upper extremity must be constantly maintained in the anticontracture position, that is, the shoulder should be kept in 90 degrees of abduction with external rotation and slight flexion by use of bedside support, sling suspension, or airplane splint.

An axilla splint (Fig. 3-2) provides support to the arm in the anticontracture

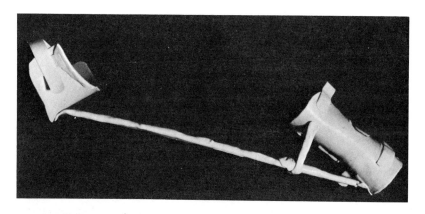

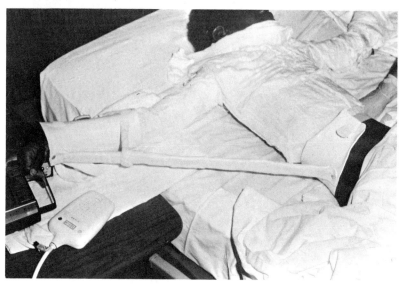

Fig. 3-2.   Axilla splint, which provides support to the arm in the anticontracture position without putting pressure over the burned area.

position without putting pressure over the injured area. This splint has an additional advantage, as it does not confine the patient to bed, but can be used to maintain arm position while the patient is ambulating. The splint is easily removed for dressing changes and exercise.

Graft/Postgraft.   During the immediate postgraft stage, the axilla splint can be continued to provide proper positioning of the upper extremity and immobilization of the graft site while allowing easy access for wound care.

Follow-Up.   After grafting, it is necessary to continue night splinting and a vigorous exercise program throughout and beyond hospitalization. Further splinting may be needed after postburn surgical reconstruction of the axilla area.

Elbow

Antecubital Fossa.   Deep second- and third-degree burns to the antecubital fossa are also noted for developing flexion contractures. This must be anticipated and dealt with appropriately in the early stage, before contracture begins.

Early Considerations.   During the critical phase, an elbow extension splint should be worn continuously and removed only for exercise or dressing changes. As the patient becomes more active and easily uses the elbow during self-care activity, the splint may be used for nighttime and rest periods only. The exercise program is stressed.

Graft/Postgraft.   After grafting, immobilization will require constant use of a splint to maintain the elbow in extension until the graft is secure. Once the graft is secure, the focus is on remobilization through exercise. The extension splint is continued to maintain the new tissue length during sleep and inactivity.

Follow-Up.   Close follow-up with continued exercise and splinting is essential, especially with children. It is extremely difficult to oppose the flexion contracture forces. The frequent need for surgical intervention must be coupled with a vigorous exercise and splinting program. Surgery is considered when the joint begins to show loss of range of motion. Multiple surgical releases may be needed to insure full joint mobility.

Posterior Surface.   Burns limited to the posterior surface of the elbow do not cause contracture and, therefore, are not usually splinted. They require elbow flexion exercises to maintain soft tissue length.

Wrist and Hand

Wrist burns are infrequently seen without associated hand burns and usually involve the extensor surface.[5] Small burns to the extensor surface of the wrist require flexion exercises. Small burns to the palmar surface require extension exercises and wrist extension position splints.

The hand is a complicated structure. It functions as a sense organ, a personalized means of communication, an aesthetic unit, and our most finely tuned functional tool. Burns to the hand can severely compromise all of these functions. Fibrosis of the edematous hand can lead to permanent deformity and loss of function.

Acute Stage (Dorsal Surface).   During the acute stage, dorsal wrist and

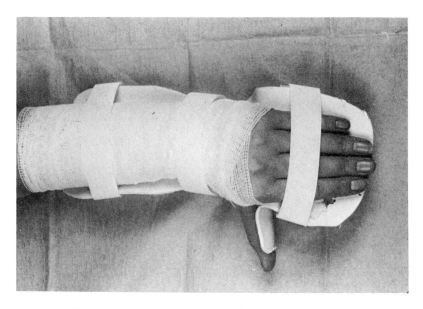

Fig. 3-3.   Hand splint for dorsal or circumferential burns.

hand burns are positioned to prevent flexion contracture. This position is 10 to 15 degrees wrist extension, 99 degrees metacarpophalangeal (MCP) flexion, and full praximal interphalangeal (PIP) and dorsal interphalangeal (DIP) extension to maintain ligament length (Fig. 3-3). Some controversy exists as to the best position for the thumb. If there are burns in or adjacent to the thenar web space, extension and abduction is the recommended position.

Circumferential burns to the hand are splinted in the position described above, but may require an increased wrist extension of 15 to 25 degrees. Early active exercise is necessary to preserve hand function. With expected extensor tendon damage, the initial flexion exercises may be performed with protective guarding at the MCP joint and gradually worked toward full fisting. Generally, if a single tendon is exposed, the therapist should continue exercise to salvage as much motion in the hand as possible.

Acute Stage (Palmar Surface).   Burns of the palmar surface of the hand are less frequently seen. If left unsplinted, these burns are prone to develop profound flexion contractures.[6] The position of splinting is similar to that previously described for dorsal burns, but with slightly less MCP flexion. The most advantageous position is 90 degrees MCP flexion, 180 degrees PIP and DIP extension. In this position, the lateral and collateral ligamentous bands are at their greatest length, minimizing potential shortening. Exercises should stress full extension of MCP joint to maintain the length of the flexor tendons.

Dynamic traction splints may be provided in later stages of healing to continue stretch to soft tissue while positioning the hand for increased function.

Postgraft Stage.   Hand splints are used during the immediate postgraft immobilization stage. These splints must provide support without direct contact on the

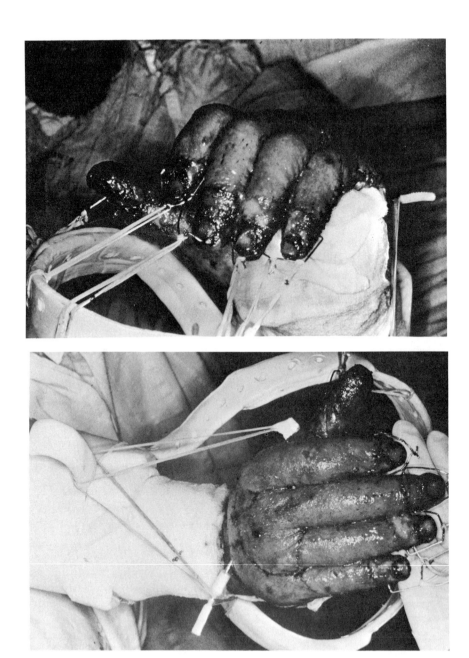

Fig. 3-4. Modified hayraker splint, which provides immobilization without direct contact on the graft site and allows for continued wound care.

graft site and allow for continued wound care. A modified hayraker splint (Fig. 3-4) can be used. This splint must be fabricated prior to surgery and applied in the operating room with the surgeon immediately after grafting. To obtain this position, the surgeon may place pins through the metacarpal to enable wrist dorsiflexion without putting pressure over the palm. Wires may be placed through the distal tufts and attached by rubberband to the outrigger to maintain PIP and DIP extension. The fingers may be removed from this device for protected active exercise.

Prolonged immobilization is poorly tolerated in the hand and may lead to permanent joint stiffness. The collateral ligaments at the MCP joint shorten with prolonged extension and, therefore, must be maintained in flexion with splints. Immobilization can cause thickening of the transverse metacarpal ligament, leading to loss of the arch of the hand. Fibrous adhesions can form over the tendons, restricting gliding movements of flexion and extension.

At the PIP joint, the soft tissues are thin and the extensor mechanism can easily be disrupted, causing an imbalance of flexion and extension, which leads to a boutonniere deformity. The collateral ligament at the PIP joint can shorten with prolonged flexion. To maintain the length of the collateral ligament, the PIP joint is positioned in extension when immobilization is needed.

Follow-Up. Once grafts are secure, exercise to maximize hand function and nighttime static hand splinting may be resumed. Dynamic splints may be used to help increase function. In Figure 3-5, a dynamic splint is used to prevent flexion contracture in the palm. The splint positions the MCP joint for improved active function. There is a hinge joint at the wrist, which allows for flexion and extension at that point.

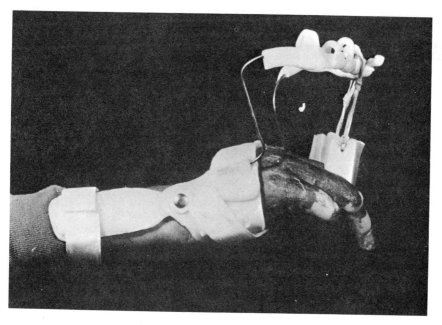

Fig. 3-5. Dynamic splint to prevent flexion contracture and improve hand function.

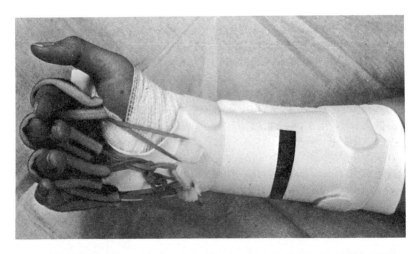

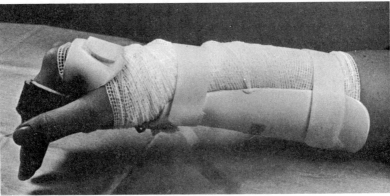

Fig. 3-6. Dynamic flexion splint. Provides slow steady stretch to maintain tissue length.

Dynamic splints may also be used to provide slow, steady stretch to maintain tissue length without inhibiting antagonistic movement. Figure 3-6 demonstrates this type of splint.

After grafting, the exercise program used to maintain joint range of motion and ligamentous and soft tissue length is continued. Activities are provided to maximize hand function. Figures 3-5 and 3-6 show activities that may be used to improve fine motor coordination and pincer grasp. The patient in these figures lacks sufficient range at the PIP joint to utilize tip-to-tip pincer grasp. In therapy, activities were designed to maximize lateral pinch for improved hand function. Activities may be provided to improve fine motor hand function (Fig. 3-7) and retrain dominance and increase muscle strength (Figs. 3-8, 3-9).

Fig. 3-7. Activities to improve pincer grasp and fine motor coordination.

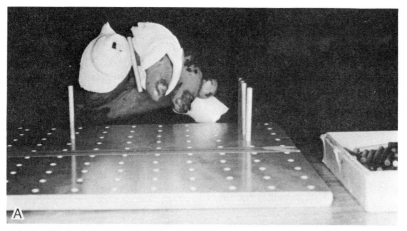

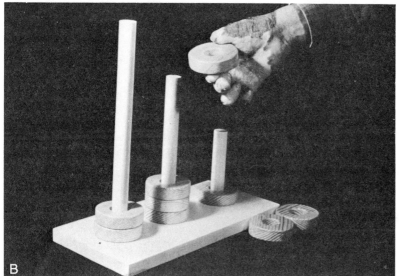

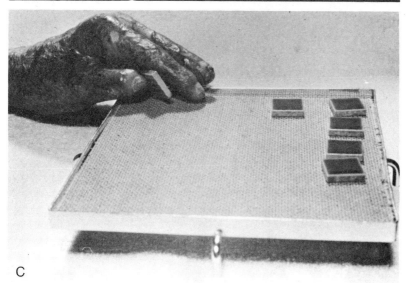

Fig. 3-7.

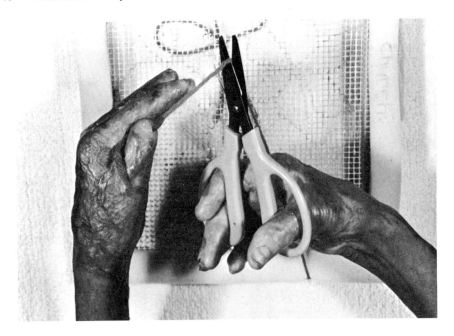

Fig. 3-8. Vocational retraining for this seamstress.

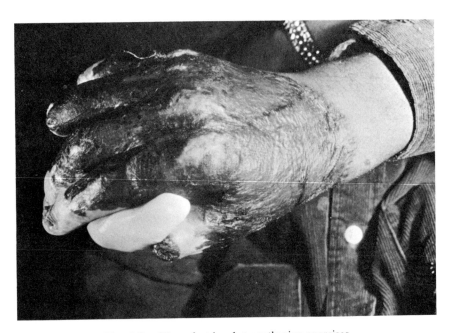

Fig. 3-9. Theraplast hand-strengthening exercises.

SPLINTING AND EXERCISE FOR THE LOWER EXTREMITY

Hips and Buttocks

Patients with burns to the hip and buttock area are placed in the prone position to eliminate pressure over the burn surface in bed during the acute and immediate postgraft stages and prior to ambulation. Once grafts are secured, the patient is encouraged to ambulate, continue range of motion exercises, and begin strengthening exercises with a physical therapist.

Popliteal Area

Deep second- and third-degree burns in the popliteal space require early splinting to prevent the development of flexion contracture. A simple posterior extension splint may be used. In Figure 3-10, the major part of the burn was on the anterior surface of the leg. Therefore, pressure of the splint with the posterior surface was

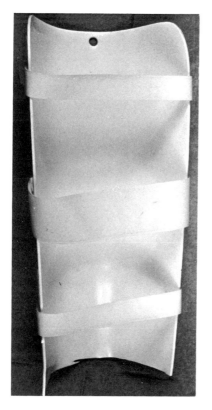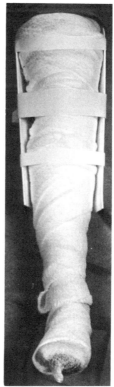

Fig. 3-10. Knee extension splint.

preferred. If rings are attached to the splint, the entire lower extremity can be elevated by attachment to overhead traction to help prevent edema.

Circumferential burns to the lower extremity may require complete elevation of the leg off the bed without applying the pressure of a splint to the burned area. This difficult position can be achieved by overhead traction attached to a Steinmann pin surgically placed in the leg.

Immediately following grafting, splints are applied to immobilize the extremity with the knee in extension. Once grafts are secure, remobilization of the knee is begun by physical therapy. Splints are used as needed to maintain range of motion.

Ankle

Burns over the posterior surface of the ankle require 90 degree dorsiflexion splints, which usually necessitates putting pressure over the burned area. This position maintains the length of the Achilles tendon. The splints should be padded, especially if used after grafting.

If ankle dorsiflexion is needed without putting pressure on the calf of the leg, a foot sandal (Fig. 3-11) can be used. This position is maintained by traction. Once the patient is ambulatory, splinting can usually be discontinued.

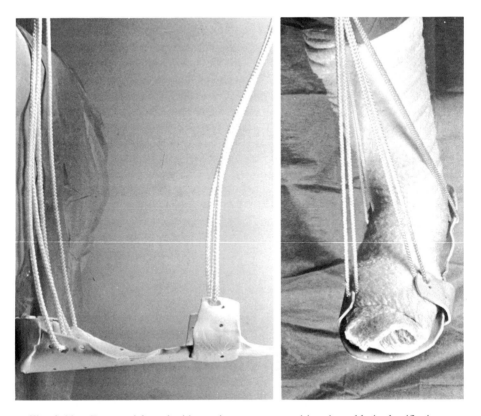

Fig. 3-11.   Foot sandal used with traction set up to position the ankle in dorsiflexion.

SPLINTING AND EXERCISES FOR THE NECK

Deep second- and third-degree burns over the anterior surface of the neck are difficult to manage. They require constant and long-term splinting and exercise to minimize the almost inevitable flexion contracture. Thus, it is important to accustom the patient to the wearing of splints as early as possible.

Early Consideration

The goal of therapy in a neck burn is to prevent flexion contracture. The method is to maintain the neck in the hyperextended position. This is done by using a cervical roll under the neck, eliminating pillows under the head, and using hyperextension splints. Hyperextension neck splints can be fabricated from low temperature thermoplastic material (Fig. 3-12). The prefabricated Philadelphia collar may also be used (Fig. 3-13). However, a custom-made splint provides a more comfortable fit with greater hyperextension. The splints are worn constantly, being removed only for dressing changes and exercise.

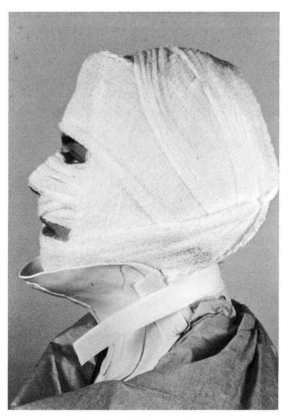

Fig. 3-12. Hyperextension neck splint fabricated from low temperature thermoplastic material.

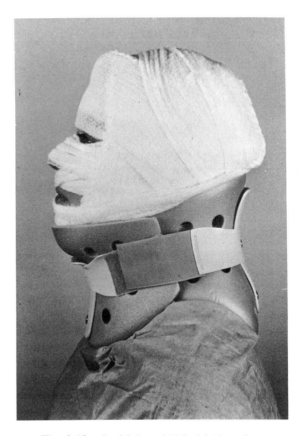

Fig. 3-13.   Prefabricated Philadelphia collar.

Active neck extension exercises are frequently performed. Static stretch is accomplished by leaning the head over the edge of the bed from the supine lying position, and utilizes gravity and the weight of the head to provide stretch.

Graft/Postgraft

During the immediate postgraft stage, the neck must be immobilized in hyperextension without placing pressure over the graft. Figure 3-14 demonstrates a type of splint used to achieve this goal. When the graft is secure, the immobilization splint is discontinued, and active exercise and static splinting is resumed. Initially, the static splint should be padded to avoid shear to the newly grafted areas. The splint is worn continuously and vigorous exercise is maintained.

Follow-Up

Unfortunately, even with long-term splinting, there is frequent recurrence of flexion contracture in the neck. This is due to the existence of strong flexor forces

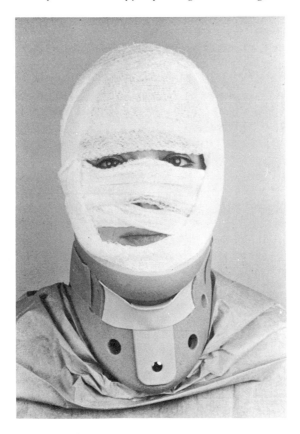

Fig. 3-13 (*Continued*).

and poor patient tolerance to long-term (three to four months) splinting. Contracture recurrence necessitates repeated surgical release and grafting. A somewhat better-tolerated splinting device is stacked rings, which are made out of cylindrical foam tubing (Fig. 3-15). This splint can be easily modified for progressive extension by the addition of more rings.

COMPRESSION

Compression is a useful adjunct in follow-up therapy. It is used to control local edema and hypertrophic scarring.[7] Once the grafts become stable, compression may be started. Adequate compression may be achieved with Ace bandages or compression garments (Fig. 3-16). If compression garments are to be used, the patient should be accurately measured as early as possible. This is usually first feasible when the edema from the injury and surgery has subsided.

The customized garment does not often deliver adequate pressure to all areas. The therapist can modify these garments to increase pressure with conformers. Con-

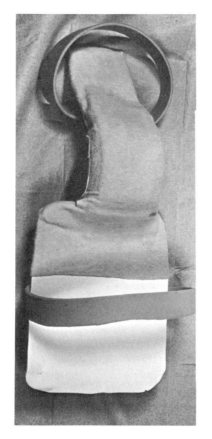
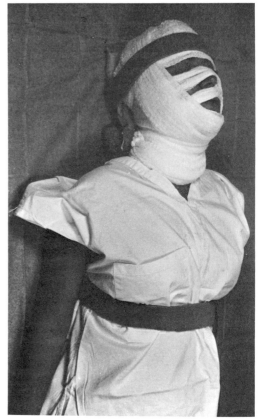

Fig. 3-14.   Postgraft hyperextension splint.

formers can be made out of foam padding, Silastic elastomer, or Otoform-K. The choice of material used depends on the specific area requiring compression and skin sensitivity. Specific problem areas that frequently require the use of conformers to achieve pressure are the cheeks, nose, palm, web spaces between the fingers, and area between the breasts.

FOLLOW-UP THERAPY

Burn wounds continue to change over a long period of time and may not reach stable maturity until many years following the accident. During this period, skin contractures may develop and require surgery. The exercise, splinting, and compression program must continue throughout this period under the careful frequent observation of the therapist. The goal is to maintain function. Exercises and activities are provided to increase range of motion, muscle strength, coordination, and to promote normal grasp patterns.

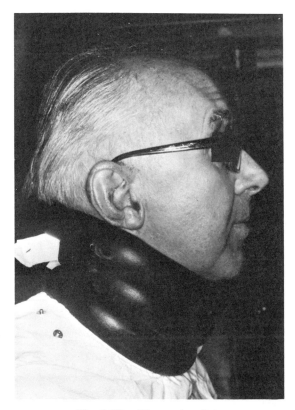

Fig. 3-15.   Ring neck splint.

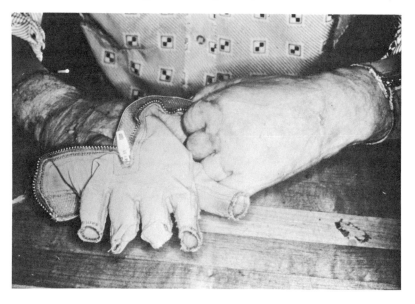

Fig. 3-16.   Jobst compression glove.

SUMMARY

The occupational therapist is an intrinsic member of the burn team. The therapist is concerned with wound management, restoration of physical function, and psychological support. The therapist is specifically involved in providing proper positioning to the injured or reconstructed part through the use of splints.

The therapy program individually designed for each patient by the occupational therapist includes the use of exercise, activities, and splinting. The program is designed to control edema and prevent the development of contractures and functional and aesthetic deformities. The program is initiated as soon as possible after admission and may continue for many years after discharge while the wounds mature.

Splinting—its rationale, materials, and application—was discussed for specific areas, as was the need for postdischarge exercise and compression garments.

REFERENCES

1. Wagner M: Care of the Burn Injured patient. Littleton: PSG , 1981
2. Bernstein NR: Emotional Care of the Facially Burned and Disfigured. Boston, Little, Brown, 1976
3. Von Prince: The Splinting of Burn Patients. Springfield, Charles C Thomas, 1974
4. Salisbury: Burns of the Upper Extremity. Philadelphia, WB Saunders, 1976
5. Sevitt S: Reactions to Injury, Burns and Their Clinical Importance. Philadelphia, JB Lippincott, 1974
6. Curtis P: The Treatment of Burns. Philadelphia, WB Saunders, 1969
7. Munster AM: Burn Care for the House Officer. Baltimore, Williams & Wilkins, 1981

4 | Exercise and Ambulation in the Burn Patient

Patricia M. Kozerefski

As medical advances increase the survival rate from severe burns, more attention must be given to the quality of life being maintained; that is, restoring the patient to his preburn physical and psychological state. This task requires the integration of skills of all members of the burn team. Foremost, the physical and occupational therapist play primary roles in maintaining and restoring the patient's optimal level of function. The therapeutic techniques incorporated into the rehabilitation program are splinting, positioning, exercise, pressure techniques, activities of daily living (ADL), and ambulation.

The purpose of this discussion is to outline the principles of exercise techniques and ambulatory activities as primary modalities in the physical rehabilitation of the burn victim. The complexities of restoring normal movement are too often overlooked in these patients, and it is the quality of movement that ultimately determines the quality of function. The effort to bring about and keep movement is as noble and difficult a task as is the effort to save the life.

EXERCISE AND AMBULATION IN THE ACUTE PHASE

Factors that Affect Movement

Impairment in motor functioning is frequently observed in the burn patient, even though in most cases no direct neurological injury has been sustained. The ability to integrate the components of movement, such as strength, endurance, coordination,

55

Table 4-1. Relation of Total Body Surface Burn to Subsequent Joint Limitation

Percent TBS Burn	Total Patients	No. with Normal Range of Motion	No. with Limited Range of Motion	Percentage with Limitation
0–10	147	135	12	8.2
10–20	139	117	22	15.8
20–30	149	107	42	28.2
30–40	107	75	32	29.9
40–50	78	42	36	46.2
50–60	38	12	26	68.4
60–70	19	5	14	73.7
70–80	3	0	3	100.0
80–90	1	0	1	100.0
90–100	0	—	—	—
Total patients	681	493	188	27.6

TBS, Total body surface.
With permission from Dobbs ER, Curreri WP: Burns: Analysis of results of physical therapy in 681 patients. J Trauma 12:242–248, 1972. © 1972 The Williams & Wilkins Co., Baltimore.

etc., is impaired. In the acute phase, the time prior to wound closure, the quality and degree of movement is affected by the extent, depth, and location of burn, as well as edema, pain, physiological imbalances, and psychological disorders. Prolonged periods of immobility and delayed initiation of physical and occupational therapy often have adverse effects.[1,2,3,4] To design and carry out an effective treatment program, it is a prerequisite to identify the way in which these factors interfere with the patient's ability to perform normal movement.

The extent to total body surface area (TBSA) burned is one factor that affects the degree of joint limitation. Dobbs and Curreri studied 681 burned patients at the Brook Army Medical Center. They found that the percent of patients with limitations in joint range of motion (ROM) increased with the extent of TBSA burned (Table 4-1).[4] It seems likely that those factors that tend to interfere with ROM are compounded in patients with larger TBSA burns.

Data collected in their study also revealed a correlation between the depth of burn and degree of joint limitation. Those patients with full-thickness (third-degree) burns sustained greater loss of joint motion than those with partial-thickness (second-degree) burns (Tables 4-2 and 4-3).[4] The physical properties of second- and third-degree burns differ during the acute phase of treatment. Prior to wound closure, the second-degree burn tissue maintains its elastic properties and is soft in texture if it remains moist. The third-degree burn is already leatherlike and inelastic prior to wound closure.[5] Therefore, it offers more resistance to movement. In addition, the granulation tissue, which starts to be laid down in the third-degree wound on approximately the third day after injury, contains the same contractile elements found in the hypertrophic scar.[6,7] These elements further increase the tissue resistance to movement. The contractile properties of the second-degree burn are more apparent after wound closure. A still deeper burn that extends into the fascial and muscle layers is

Table 4-2. Area of Third-Degree Burn and
Percent of Limitation

Joint	Total Burned	Total with Limitation	Percent
Hand	309	137	44.3
Elbow	306	107	35.0
Shoulder	160	87	54.4
Cervical	40	24	60.0
Foot	90	14	15.5
Knee	287	42	14.6
Total	1,192	411	34.5

With permission from Dobbs ER, Cureri WP:
Burns: Analysis of results of physical therapy in
681 patients. J Trauma 12:242–248, 1974. © 1972
The Williams & Wilkins Co., Baltimore.

characteristically charred, inelastic, and even more limited in its ability to allow
movement.

The location and configuration of a burn in relation to the underlying joint axis
and adjacent body parts will affect the patient's ability to move in particular direc-
tions. Generally, those movements that stretch the involved tissue are the most difficult to perform. (The specific effects that the location and configuration of the burn
have on determining the position of deformity will be discussed in detail later.)

Edema formation resulting from increased capillary permeability and the subsequent accumulation of protein-rich fluid in the extracellular compartment restricts
blood and lymphatic flow,[8] and joint motion. This happens particularly in the digits
of the hand and in large areas of deep circumferential burns, where there is limited
space to allow for the edema. Prolonged edema contributes to the laying down of
fibrin, which coupled with immobilization contributes to the formation of adhesions,
disrupting the normal sliding and gliding motion between the underlying structures.
If appropriate measures are not taken, secondary changes in the articular and sup-

Table 4-3. Area Second-Degree Burn and Percent
of Limitation

Joint	Total Burned	Total with Limitation	Percent
Hand	603	33	5.5
Elbow	554	23	4.2
Shoulder	428	27	6.3
Cervical	161	4	2.5
Foot	49	6*	12.2
Knee	325	5	1.5
Total	2,120	98	4.6

*In two patients, one with CNS involvement
and one with bilateral peroneal nerve injuries, limitation was not due to the burn.

With permission from Dobbs ER, Curreri WP:
Burns: Analysis of results of physical therapy in
681 patients. J Trauma 12:242–248, 1972.

porting structures will result in joint stiffness and decreased joint excursion. The degree of limitation is adversely affected by increasing age and duration of immobilization. Permanent interphalangeal joint stiffness has been reported as early as two weeks after burn injury in patients over 15 years of age who experienced both edema and prolonged immobilization.[1,2,9,10,11]

Pain and the patient's tolerance to pain will affect his capacity to move. Superficial second-degree burns are hypersensitive to temperature, exposure to air, and light touch, whereas deeper second-degree burns are less sensitive.[12] Although third-degree burns are generally described as being insensitive due to the destruction of cutaneous nerve endings, patients with third-degree burns often do complain about pain. The pain may raise from interspersed areas of second-degree burn or from the perimeter of the third-degree burn, which is often an area of second-degree interface. Therefore, movement of a body part with a third-degree burn generally elicits pain. In order to avoid pain or in anticipation of avoiding pain associated with movement, the patient immobilizes the involved part in a position of comfort resembling the fetal position. This position is often maintained by muscle cocontraction or self-splinting. When asked to move the involved body part actively, the patient may have difficulty in voluntarily releasing tone within the antagonistic muscle group and in moving beyond the limits of his pain threshold.

Changes in the patient's mental functioning due to physiological or psychological stresses and impairments can affect the patient's motor control. CP Artz describes: "The main psychological complication in the first two or three weeks after injury is delirium. It is characterized by major impairment of thinking, memory, and perception. The symptoms that accompany delirium, such as hallucinations, delusions, apathy, agitation, and withdrawal, may mimic other psychiatric disorders. Usually, the patient is worse at night and better during the daytime. Physiological factors such as infection, hypoxia, metabolic imbalances, and cardiovascular insufficiency are most important. Only after having ruled out all these possibilities can one resort to psychological explanations for delirium, such as sensory input overload, delirium, or sleep deprivation."[3]

Regardless of the etiology, delirium and other psychological impairments may affect the patient's ability to perform voluntary or directed movement. For example, the patient may not be able to follow a simple command such as "lift up your arm." In more severe cases, varying degrees of muscle hypertonicity, tremor, and ataxia may result.[13]

Prolonged periods of immobility or delayed onset of an exercise program may contribute to musculoskeletal and cardiovascular alterations. Bone structures that are not stressed through activity soon become demineralized and osteoporotic. Muscle atrophy (weakness) results from disuse due to the breakdown of protein structures within that tissue.[14,15] Alterations in the efficiency of the cardiovascular system for oxygen uptake, cardiac output, stroke volume, and heart rate following prolonged periods of bedrest have been described by Saltin et al.[16]

Those factors outlined above that interfere with the quality and degree of movement are generally compounded as the extent and degree of burn increases. Their adverse effects on the patient's ability to move can be prevented or minimized if a purposefully designed and executed exercise program is initiated early after injury.

Factors that Affect the Exercise Program

During the acute phase, an aggressive exercise program that incorporates the components of strength, endurance, rhythm, dexterity, etc., should ensure maintenance of function. However, as the percent of TBSA burn increases, so does the body's response increase, affecting the function of multiple-organ systems. This response is compounded in children, the aged, and those patients with preexisting medical complications. The capacity to perform varying degrees of exercise and activity depends upon the normal and interrelated functioning of the body's systems.[17] Even following adequate resuscitation, the existing increased physiologic demands, metabolic alterations, and decreased reserve as a result of the thermal injury may not allow the body to accommodate to an optimal exercise program. In view of the above, the following should be considered before designing the exercise program.

Immediately following injury, the body shifts fluid from the vascular compartment to the extravascular space. Therefore the patient becomes hypovolemic. Cardiac output drops dramatically immediately postinjury, reaches normal values within 36 hours, and subsequently exceeds normal values. Oxygen consumption increases. Pulmonary insufficiency may develop as a result of inhalation injury, pulmonary edema, or airway obstruction. Hyperventilation may result from metabolic acidosis or cardiac insufficiency. The constituents and the flow of blood alters. The resting metabolic rate in a burn up to 40 to 50 percent TBSA increases linearly, leveling off in the larger percent TBSA burns, and declines with wound closure. Environmental, psychological, and physical stresses, such as changes in room temperature, infection, and fear, will further increase metabolic demands.[8,18,19,20,21]

Carter et al. conducted a study on 10 control and 10 burned male subjects between the ages of 18 and 33 that measured the oxygen consumption (VO_2) in both groups at rest and following straight-leg raising and short-arc quadriceps femoris muscle exercises. A significantly higher resting VO_2 was recorded in the burn subjects. In addition, the burn subjects used significantly more oxygen to perform both sets of exercises. The comparison of the mean change from resting VO_2 to exercise VO_2 between both groups was insignificant.

In this study the maximum VO_2 recorded in the burn subjects did not reach the upper limits of oxygen uptake required for light work, but these subjects did begin exercising at a significantly higher VO_2 than the control subjects.[22] Consequently, during the acute phase the exercises must be designed to achieve the patient's functional needs while minimizing stress.[23] At this time, the primary goal of the exercise program is to maintain simple range of motion, not to maintain or develop existing muscle mass, particularly at the ends of the range of motion.[24] This will ensure complete joint excursion, prevent the onset of contractures in the damaged and underlying tissues, and maintain a foundation on which a progressive exercise program can be based.

Selecting the Appropriate Method of Exercises

Active exercise is the preferred type of exercise during the acute phase, although active assistive, passive, isometric, and resistive exercises may play a role. When executed appropriately, active exercise serves to meet the patient's functional, physiological, and psychological needs with minimal stress to the patient.

Movement controlled by active muscle contraction allows for normal articular excursion and for normal tension length ratio of the supporting musculoskeletal structures. Active movement helps maintain muscle mass (strength) by aiding in the restoration of protein structures within the muscle tissue, which are depleted by the increased metabolic demands and prolonged periods of inactivity.[23] Movement elicits proprioceptive, motor, and sensory feedback, which helps reinforce purposeful movement. The direct effect of active exercise on edema remains controversial, although it is generally agreed upon that prolonged immobilization coupled with edema contributes to venous and lymphatic stasis.[9] Active exercise aids in venous and lymphatic return, and by improving circulation decreases the risk of thromboemboli.[25] Participating in an active exercise program also helps the patient's emotional wellbeing by reinforcing his capacity to move independently.[24]

It may be necessary to implement active assistive exercises when the patient cannot independently achieve the end of the range of motion. This will require hands-on techniques to overcome the resistance of the contractile nature of the involved tissue or the underlying muscle tone in the antagonistic muscle groups. Care must be taken not to turn an active assistive program into a session of overzealous passive exercise or a resistive battle with the patient. Active assistive exercises are also indicated for those patients who cannot tolerate an active exercise program due to decreased cardiac reserve, poor ventilation, and increased metabolic demands.

Passive exercises have historically been discouraged at this time in the treatment of the burn patient. Although passive exercise requires less energy expenditure, it does not fulfill as many of the patient's needs as judicious active exercise. If performed too aggressively and poorly, the articular surfaces can be traumatized. Overzealous passive exercise in the form of quick, jerky movements beyond tissue resistance will result in microscopic or visible tissue tears and bleeding, and will ultimately facilitate scarring and contracture formation.[26] The key to incorporating slow, gentle, passive exercise into the program designed to obtain the full ranges lies within the therapist's technique and ability to differentiate between the elastic properties of burned and underlying tissue and the point of tissue resistance. This is particularly significant when performing slow, gentle, passive exercise on the patient who is comatose or under anesthesia.[27] With no response from the patient, the therapists must rely on skill and their own sensory feedback to gauge the upper limits of tissue extensibility.

Resistive exercises may be contraindicated during the acute phase of treatment in relationship to the extent TBSA burned and the patient's medical status. Certainly, a healthy young adult who sustained less than a 15 percent TBSA burn with no inhalation insult could tolerate a resistive exercise program to maintain strength, because there is sufficient reserve to accommodate to the stress. An elderly or adolescent patient with the same percentage of burned TBSA may not be able to do so. Resistive exercises should be avoided in all patients with larger percent burns because of the increased metabolic demand placed on the patient as a result of the thermal injury. The use of neurological inhibitory and facilitory techniques such as contract-relax or rhythmic initiation incorporate a resistive component, and therefore they should be used cautiously during the acute phase of treatment. It should also be realized that a patient who is fighting against the therapist's attempts to perform assistive or passive exercise is indeed performing resistive exercise.

The selection of the method of exercise most appropriate to meet the total needs of the patient must be carefully evaluated. Although active exercise is preferred, modifications in the selection of the method of exercise is indicated when there are changes in the patient's medical as well as functional status. Daily evaluation of the patient's response to the exercise program is imperative in order to detect changes in the patient's performance, to identify the underlying cause affecting those changes, and to appropriately modify the exercise program to meet the patient's needs.

Designing and Carrying Out the Exercise Program

An understanding of the dynamics that affect the position of contracture or deformity is necessary in order to design an effective exercise program. The following factors in combination will influence the ultimate position of contracture: the contractile nature of the involved tissue; the extent, location, and configuration of burn; the patient's resting position of comfort; and the relative strength of the underlying muscle mass.

Possible deformities due to the contractile nature of the involved tissue should be anticipated. Burned tissue may contract or shorten during the healing process. The contractile forces of the burned tissue can be so strong as to dislocate the smaller joints, as those in the hand. In order to determine the direction of forces exerted by the burned tissue, the extent, location, and configuration of the burn relative to the underlying and adjacent body parts should be assessed. For example, is the burn wound anterior or posterior to the underlying joint axis? does it spiral around the long axis of the extremity? is it circumferential? does it bridge the joint? is it spotty? how close is it to adjacent uninvolved joints? The forces applied by the burned tissue, however, may not be great enough to overcome the position the patient assumes for comfort. Therefore, in some instances the burn tissue may be maintained in an elongated position. The position of deformity may also be affected by the difference in the relative strength of the underlying muscle masses. For example, the elbow flexors are stronger than the elbow extensors; therefore, there is a predisposition toward elbow flexion contractures.

Depending on the patient, any one of these factors can become the dominant force in influencing the ultimate position of contracture. For example, a burn over the posterior aspect of the elbow will probably not result in an elbow extension contracture because the relative strength of the elbow flexors is greater than the elbow extensors, and elbow flexion is the position of comfort the patient would be likely to assume if left to his own devices. With a burn over the anterior aspect of the elbow, the anticipated position of deformity would be elbow flexion for the same reasons. The predisposition for the position of contracture of certain body parts have been determined by Dobbs and Curreri (Table 4-4).[4]

Once the anticipated direction of deformity has been identified, the direction of counterforces to be applied can be determined. In order to minimize stress the direction of the exercise should be antagonistic to the direction of the anticipated deformity, and should concentrate on those motions that are most difficult to maintain. The

Table 4-4. Predisposition to and Prevention of Contracture

Joint	Degree of Burn	Predisposition	Prevention
Hand	2° and 3°	Flexion of wrist	Extension; no wrist deviation
		Adduction of thumb	Radial abduction and opposition
	2°	Varies; position of comfort	Complete range and function of all joints
	3°	Hyperextension of metacarpophalangeal (MP) joints	Flexion of MPs to 90°, wrist in extension
		Flexion of proximal interphalangeal (PIP) joints	Extension with MP joints in flexion
Elbow*	2° and 3°	Pronation and flexion	Full supination with both extension and flexion; emphasize extension
Shoulder*	2° and 3°	Adduction	Full flexion (occasionally also full abbduction)
Anterior cervical area	2° and 3°	Flexion	Hyperextension
Knee	2° and 3°	Flexion	Full extension
Foot*	2° and 3°	Plantar flexion	Dorsiflexion; foot in neutral position

*Predisposition exists without surface burns.

With permission from Dobbs ER, Curreri WP: Burns: Analysis of results of physical therapy in 681 patients. J Trauma 12:242–248, 1972. © 1972 The Williams & Wilkins Co., Baltimore.

number of repetitions of exercise should be proportional to the degree of anticipated contracture, while considering the patient's tolerance. Some patients can achieve full ROM on their first attempt. Others will require five or more repetitions to attain full ROM or their maximum available ROM. Increasing the number of repetitions of the exercise, as well as adding an assistive component, can help to restore ROM that has been lost by tissue contracture. Patients who require extended exercise programs but who have limited tolerance may respond better to multiple short bouts of exercise throughout the course of the day. If the patient's tolerance allows it, movements should be multiaxial to obtain a maximum stretch of the involved and underlying tissues, while attempting to obtain the end ranges of the involved and adjacent joints.

Additional stresses associated with carrying out an exercise program can be minimized by simple measures. Anxieties and fears not only increase the patient's metabolic needs by increasing his emotional stress but also lower the patient's tolerance to pain.[28] Explaining the purpose of the program, reassuring the patient, and establishing a rapport should decrease anxieties about exercising, as well as motivate the patient. Stress associated with pain or the anticipation of pain on movement may manifest itself by increased muscle tension and cocontraction. The exercise program can be preceded with a brief period using relaxation techniques, hypnosis, or biofeedback to reduce this tension. Although these techniques require extra time and patience, the end result usually justifies the effort.

Some patients prefer to exercise while submerged in a whirlpool or Hubbard tank because the water softens the eschar and tends to be relaxing.[29,30] Other patients associate tank time with wound debridement and pain. Therefore, they find it difficult to exercise at that time and prefer to exercise at the bedside or on the rehabilitation unit. Attempting to perform exercises at a time when the patient is being stressed by or preoccupied with other procedures is usually futile. Each patient should be evaluated individually as to his need for pain-relieving medication prior to the exercise session.

The outcome of the exercise session can be enhanced and the stress reduced in the patient who is cooperative and motivated. Patients usually express their opposition to exercise by being verbally abusive and physically combative. Attempts at performing exercises while the patient is expressing this behavior creates frustration for the therapist as well as the patient. If the patient does not respond to explanations of the rationale for exercising, more carefully planned and consistently executed methods for motivation must be employed. This is particularly important when working with children. A simple method is making a contract with the patient. For example, offer him some control of the program by allowing him to select the treatment time. Be emphatic, however, that you will treat him at that time with the understanding that he must participate in the entire program. Offering the patient tokens that will satisfy other needs may be effective. As an example, offer to bring a patient to an area where he can have a cigarette if he is allowed and if that is his need.

A most difficult motivation technique employs behavior modification. This requires a degree of consistency on the part of all team members, which is difficult to expect in the hospital environment. One successful form of behavior modification is rewarding the patient with ''stroking'' or positive feedback when his behavior is favorable. The use of bedside graphs and charts to indicate the patient's progress is helpful, particularly when the patient can map out his progress himself.

It is important not to totally abandon the uncooperative and unmotivated patient. These patients often do not understand the possible repercussions of being noncompliant with the rehabilitation program. If handled properly, they usually accept at least part of the treatment regime.

The significance of exercising will have its major impact on the patient when it relates to his ability to perform self-care activities. Not only do such activities give a means of measuring progress, but they also provide the patient with a sense of independence in an environment in which he has little control. From a therapeutic point of view, self-care activities reinforce functional carryover of the exercise program by encouraging integration of the components of movement and providing sensory, proprioceptive, and motor stimulation.

When the patient is medically stable, he should be expected to participate in grooming and self-care activities. A basin equipped with toothbrush, comb, and soap, should be issued to each patient and a time set aside in the morning for the patient to carry out his own grooming activities. Those who are able to do so should be encouraged to don their own hospital gowns and slippers. The more mobile patient can take the responsibility for tidying the environment in their hospital rooms. All patients should participate in self-feeding activities.

Often patients will face difficulties and become impatient when attempting to complete these tasks, particularly those with hand burns. Forcing a patient to complete a task which is beyond his capabilities will lead to further frustration and discourage further attempts to perform independent tasks. The therapist must take time to realistically evaluate the patient's ability and performance in order to determine the possible need for adaptive equipment. For example, patients with hand burns often require assistance in organizing their meal trays, but then can feed themselves independently with the aid of built-up or long-handled eating utensils, universal cuffs, plate guards, sandwich holders, and cup holders. As the patient progresses it is necessary to discourage adaptive aids in order to encourage independence.

Family members and friends of the patient often feel they are being helpful when they assist the patient in ADL and feeding. They must be made to understand that assisting a patient who is capable of completing a task independently only reinforces the patient's feeling of helplessness and undermines rehabilitative efforts.

Progressing the Exercise Program

During the later stages of the acute phase of treatment, the body's systems generally begin to function more normally. The patient's improving medical status allows the therapist to modify and advance the exercise program. Assessing the patient's medical status daily and communicating with the medical staff will offer the therapist information about the patient's increased tolerance. This is a critical time in the rehabilitation program. Those factors previously outlined that interfered with the patient's motor abilities are resolving, and a true picture of the patient's functional capabilities emerges.

Regardless of whether or not the patient exhibits complete ROM, he may have difficulty performing smooth coordinated functional movement within the available ROM. Movements that require simultaneous motions of more than one joint are difficult. The rotational component of movement necessary for function is omitted. In addition, the patient exhibits difficulty moving in diagonal planes. For example, a patient with upper extremity burns who has good ROM may have difficulty reaching across the table to pick up a full cup and bring it to his mouth. Attempts to integrate speed or rhythm into a movement pattern is difficult for the burn patient and often results in a gross distortion of the movement.

It is appropriate at this time to consider the second objective of the exercise program; that is, to improve the quality of movement within the available range. While straight ROM exercises should continue as part of the program to restore lost ROM or to prevent potential contractures, the program should begin to involve more gross body parts, such as an extremity, hand and neck, or trunk. One should then progress to include combinations of uninvolved and involved body parts, such as bilateral upper or lower extremities, upper extremities and trunk, and ipsilateral extremities. These patterns of movement should be coordinated and multiaxial, and should include a rotary component. Performing the movements at varied speeds and rhythms will provide the patient with the previously deprived sensory, proprioceptive, and motor stimulation. The diagonal patterns of movement described by Knott and Voss are ideal for meeting the objectives of the program at this time.[31]

At the time of wound closure, more of a resistive component can be incorporated into the exercise program. Initially, resistance may only be used in facilitory fashion such as contract-relax or repeated contractions. Later on, one should progress to a strengthening program of the muscle groups that are antagonistic to the direction of contracture. General conditioning programs usually begin after the patient is discharged from the hospital.

Special Considerations

Modifying and grading the exercise program is also dependent upon the status of the burn wound. Areas of newly applied autographs, exposed tendons, and exposed joints will require special attention.

In order to ensure good graft take, newly grafted areas are immobilized in a functional position for a period of three to five days. The physical therapy program resumes with gentle active exercises and progresses as the integrity of the graft improves. Shearing forces on the newly healed graft should be avoided while exercising.

Areas of exposed tendons have historically been immobilized through the use of splints or internal fixation to avoid overstretching and resultant tearing of the tendon. When joint fusion is not preferred, this author has safely executed gentle active exercises to areas of exposed tendons in attempts to avoid joint stiffness. The tendon is first placed on maximum slack by appropriately positioning the joints over which the tendon bridges. Individual underlying joints may be actively exercised if the tendon is maintained in a shortened position and the movement does not create significant tension in that tendon.

Burn wounds that extend to the joint capsule or into the joint will require prolonged periods of immobilization to adequately preserve or restore the integrity of the joint and supporting structures. Surgical intervention through the application of autografts or flaps is often necessary. Starting an exercise program for areas of exposed joints should be carefully discussed and planned with the physician. In more severe cases, joint fusion in a functional position is indicated.[32 s,33]

Ambulation

Early ambulation is an essential part of the rehabilitation program whether or not the patient has burns on the lower extremities. It decreases the risk of thromboemboli, helps maintain ROM and strength in the lower extremities, and provides the patient with a sense of functional independence. Recommendations for the timing of ambulation activities vary from beginning on the day of admission to two or three times a shift, three days after admisson. Generally, each patient's medical status should be individually evaluated to determine his tolerance for such a demanding activity. Patients with catheters, I.V.'s, and cardiac monitors, and even those on respirators are not necessarily excluded as candidates for ambulation, as long as they are medically stable and have enough reserve to tolerate the activity. With such patients, more planning time will be required to organize the environment prior to standing or ambulating.

Prior to ambulation, the burned lower extremity must first be provided with elastic bandage support to prevent venous stasis and edema. Often the vascular network within the involved tissue does not respond to normal vasomotor control.[34] If the patient stands without elastic bandage support, purple discoloration and bleeding may be evident in the unhealed, healed, or grafted areas. Therefore, it is recommended that elastic bandages be applied to the involved lower extremities while the patient is still in the recumbent position. Uninvolved lower extremities may also

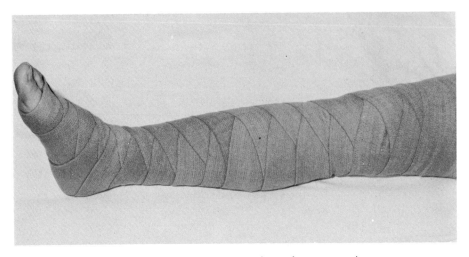

Fig. 4-1.   Elastic bandage wrapping to lower extremity.

require elastic support.[35] Even with the use of elastic supports, prolonged periods of dependency should be avoided. Lower extremity evaluation is recommended between standing activities.

The wounds should be properly managed prior to wrapping them with the elastic bandages. First, topical antimicrobial agents or burn wound dressings are applied. Next comes a layer of nonadherent dressings over the wounds to allow for ease and comfort when removing the bandages. A single layer of Kerlix or the like should cover the nonadherent dressings. Finally, the elastic bandages can be applied. Begin around the ball of the foot and proceed proximally, wrapping in a figure eight pattern. Each wrap should be one inch apart. All areas should be covered and wrinkles avoided to prevent venous stasis (Fig. 4-1). For those patients with burns on the toes, the bandage should include the toes. A soft, padded cast boot may be indicated for patients with burns on the plantar surface of the foot.

The patient will respond better if he has a clear understanding of what he is about to do and what is expected of him. Reassurance and encouragement will help alleviate his anxieties and provide a motivating force.

The patient should be encouraged to come to the sitting position at the edge of the bed with minimal assistance from the nurse, overhead trapeze, or the therapist. Although this will take more time, these activities require the patient to use many components of movement and to integrate motor planning skills in order to complete the task. Once the patient is dangling at the edge of the bed, he may be reluctant to stand because of the increased pain in his lower extremities from dependency and the fear that they may not be able to support his body weight. Patience and reassurance on the part of the staff may encourage the patient to complete a standing pivot transfer into a nearby chair. It may be necessary to supply the patient with a walker or other assistive devices to alleviate his fear of falling. To obtain maximal benefit from the activity and to discourage long-term dependency on their use, unnecessary assistive devices should be avoided. Those patients with orthostatic hypotension may have to begin on a carefully monitored progressive tilt table program before attempting ambulation activities.

As the patient gains confidence and tolerance to activity improves, a more progressive ambulation program can be considered. This next step is to increase the distance of ambulation and improve the quality of the gait. Patients often exhibit an antalgic gait, characterized by flexion at the knees, hips, and trunk (Fig. 4-2). Emphasizing a heel-to-toe gait pattern with equal-step lengths, reciprocal body motions, and good body alignment will help to maintain the quality of the gait and to prevent long-term postural changes. Heel cord stretching exercises should be performed during gait activities.

The use of mirrors will provide the patient with visual feedback about postural and gait deviations. Exercise equipment, such as a restorator, bicycle, or kinetron may be indicated for some patients in maintaining and improving lower extremity functioning during the acute phase of treatment.

The grafted lower extremity requires special consideration. For areas grafted below the knee, dependency should be avoided for a period of approximately ten days after grafting. Standing activities will require Ace bandage support as previously described. It is best to begin with short bouts of ambulation, followed by lower

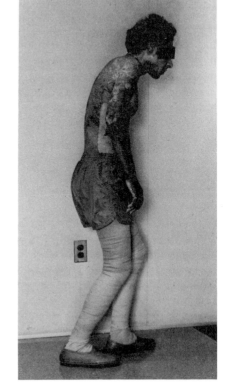

Fig. 4-2. Typical flexed posture during ambulation.

extremity elevation, and progress to longer periods of dependency while frequently monitoring the integrity and appearance of the autograft. When purple discoloration or bleeding is evident, the lower extremity should be elevated.

EXERCISE IN THE CHRONIC PHASE

In the chronic phase or postrecovery period (the time after wound closure), movement is generally impaired by existing contractures and the dynamic contractile nature of the hypertrophic scar. Pressure materials and sustained traction applied by splints aid in improving range of motion by remodeling scar tissue. Exercising will help maximize these effects and improve functional ability.

The program must first be directed at maintaining or restoring complete elongation of the scar tissue over isolated joints. This will allow complete joint excursion, thereby maintaining the integrity of the articular surfaces and the tension length ratios of the supporting musculoskeletal structure. In addition, obtaining maximal elongation of the scar tissue should be considered by assessing the effects the location and shape of the scar has on the patient's ability to perform simultaneous movements of adjacent joints and body parts. For example, a patient with a healed upper extremity burn that extends over the axilla and onto the trunk may obtain complete elbow extension when the arm is resting at the side of the trunk. However, as the patient abducts his arm, he may be unable to maintain complete elbow extension due to the total stretch being placed on the contracted scar tissue (Figs. 4-3 and 4-4).

Attempts to achieve complete ROM should begin with active exercises immediately after the removal of the pressure garments or splints in order to take advan-

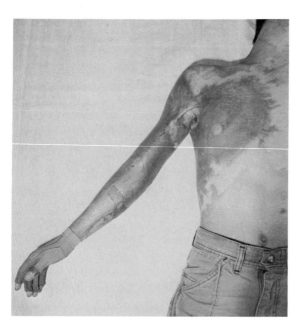

Fig. 4-3. Patient with healed right upper extremity and trunk burns exhibits loss of elbow extension as the shoulder is abducted owing to the maximum stretch being placed on the scar tissue.

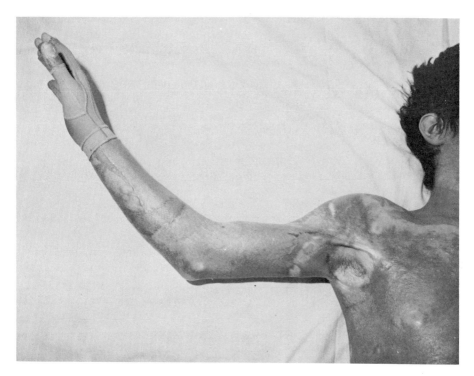

Fig. 4-4. Patient with healed right upper extremity and trunk burns exhibits loss of elbow extension as the shoulder is abducted, owing to the maximum stretch being placed on the scar tissue.

tage of their effects. Clinical changes in the scar tissue can occur quickly after their removal.[36] In full ROM is not achieved, efforts have to be made to identify the cause of the problem. When pain and subsequent muscle cocontraction are hindering the patient's ability to complete the range, neurophysiological facilitory or inhibitory techniques aimed at encouraging agonistic muscle contractions may be indicated. The patient might also respond to relaxation techniques. Persistent or acute joint pain may be indicative of other complications, such as ectopic bone formation, and should be ruled out before progressing with the exercise program.[37,38] Joint stiffness caused by prolonged periods of immobility can be appropriately treated with joint mobilization techniques. When the limitations are caused by the contractile forces of the scar tissue, the method of exercise must be modified to effectively improve ROM.

Slow, sustained stretching of the scar to the point of tissue blanching has proven to be effective in elongating the scar. It can be applied manually by the therapist, through gravity, or through the use of assistive devices such as pulleys or traction units.[39]

The effectiveness of the exercise program, whether active or passive (slow, sustained stretching, or traction), can be enhanced if the treatment is preceded by the application of skin lubricants, mild heat, paraffin, or the use of ultrasound.

The application of skin lubricants decreases itching and improves skin pliability by decreasing dryness. Attempting to exercise a dry surface may lead to painful cracking of the tissue and ultimately facilitate some loss of ROM. Only a light application of lubricant is recommended.

The application of paraffin as described by Head and Helm proved effective in increasing the obtainable ROM. Not only does it act as a lubricating agent because of the mineral oil content, but it also offers the physiological effects of mild heat.

The use of whirlpools as an adjunctive modality is discouraged during this time of the recovery period, as it is an ineffective heating modality within the safe temperature limits recommended for healed burns, and can lead to skin dryness.[38]

The physiological and clinical effects of ultrasound on the scar tissue is not well-documented in the literature. Johnson et al. have described its heating effects as increasing the extensibility of connective tissue and recommend its use in conjunction with sustained stretching.[40]

When maximum increases in ROM have been achieved during each exercise session, the emphasis of the program should shift to improving functional ability and encouraging general body conditioning. This part of the program should include a period of hands-on mat activities as well as use of exercise equipment, such as exercise balls, pulleys, bicycles, treadmills, and so on. The goals of the program should be directed to the long-term needs of the patient. For example, a patient who is considering work as a construction worker will require a more intensive conditioning program than a patient who returns to sedentary work.

All patients should be encouraged to carry out a home exercise program and perform or attempt to perform ADL independently. The use of adaptive equipment should be used with discretion when the patient cannot carry out an activity independently.

To ensure maintenance or restoration of optimal functional levels, the patient

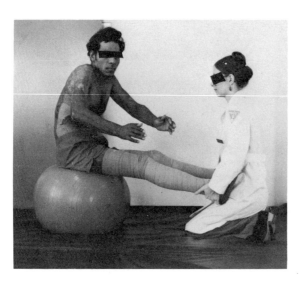

Fig. 4-5. Patient exercising on the Swedish ball to improve balance, coordination, and trunk rotation.

should continue on an exercise program until the time of scar tissue maturation. After discharge from the hospital, the more involved patient may require daily outpatient therapy appointments or admission to a rehabilitation facility. On the other hand, the patient may leave the hospital with good ROM and function and develop gross limitations after the time of discharge. Therefore, close monitoring of the patient's functional status is imperative until complete scar tissue maturation is achieved. When losses in ROM are noted, immediate therapeutic intervention is required. As the scar tissue matures and the patient's functional status improves, the intensity of the therapeutic program can decrease.

Even with frequent and vigorous therapeutic intervention, limitations in ROM cannot always be avoided. Although reconstructive surgery may eventually be necessary, the therapist and patient must remain committed to the exercise program. Maintaining the available ROM will help to minimize the extent of the reconstructive surgery. Maintaining muscle strength within the available range will improve the probability of a good functional outcome after surgery.

ACKNOWLEDGMENT

I would like to thank Dr. Willibald Nagler, Ms. Joy Cordery, Ms. Christine Khaleeli, Ms. Elaine Sandel, and other members of the Rehabilitation team for their contributions to this chapter.

REFERENCES

1. Dobbs ER: Physical therapy. pp 492–499. In: Burns A Team Approach, eds. Artz CP, Moncrief JA, Pruitt BA. Philadelphia, WB Saunders, 1979
2. Salisbury RE, Loveless S, Silverstein P, Wilmore DW, Moylan JA, Pruitt BA: Postburn edema of the upper extremity: evaluation of present treatment. J Trauma 13:857–862, 1973
3. Artz CP: Psychological considerations. pp 461–465. In: Burns A Team Approach, eds. Artz CP, Moncrief JA, Pruitt BA. Philadelphia, WB Saunders, 1979
4. Dobbs ER, Curreri WP: Burns: analysis of results of physical therapy in 681 patients. J Trauma 12:242–248, 1972
5. Artz CP: The body's response to heat. pp 23–44. In: Burns A Team Approach, eds. Artz CP, Moncrief JA Pruitt BA. Philadelphia, WB Saunders, 1979
6. Baur PS, Parks DH, Larson DL: The healing of burn wounds. Clins Plast Surg 4:389–407, 1977
7. Gabbiani G, Hirschel BJ, Ryan GB: Granulation tissue as a contractile organ. J Exp Med 135:719–734, 1972
8. Baxter CP: Fluid volume and electrolyte changes of the early postburn period. Clin Plast Surg 1:693–709, 1974
9. Peacock EE, Madden JW, Trier WC: Some studies on the treatment of burned hands. Ann Surg 171:903–914, 1970
10. Peacock EE: Some biochemical and biophysical aspects of joint stiffness: role of collagen synthesis as opposed to altered molecular bonding. Ann Surg 164:1–12, 1966
11. Habal MB: The burned hand: a planned treatment program. J Trauma 18:587–595, 1978

12. Moncrief JA: The body's response to heat. pp 23–44. In: Burns A Team Approach, eds. Artz CP, Moncrief JA, Pruitt BA. Philadelphia, WB Saunders, 1979
13. Engel GL, Romano J: Delirium, a syndrome of cerebral insufficiency. J Chron Dis 9:260–277, 1959
14. Abramson AS: Exercise in paraplegia. p 747. In: Therapeutic Exercise, ed. Licht S. Baltimore, Waverly Press, 1965
15. Astrand P, Rodahl K: Textbook of Work Physiology. New York, McGraw-Hill, 1977
16. Saltin B, Blomqist JH, Mitchell JH, Johnson RL, Wildenthal K, Chapman CB: Response to submaximal and maximal exercise after bedrest and training. Circulation 38 (Suppl. 7), 1968
17. Littell EH: Support responses of the cardiovascular system to exercise. Phys Ther 61:1260–1264, 1981
18. Moylan JA, Alexander LG: Diagnosis and treatment of inhalation injury. World J Surg 2:185–191, 1978
19. Pruitt BA, Flemma RJ, Oivincenti FC, Foley FD, Mason AD: Pulmonary complications in burn patients. J Thorac Cardiovasc Surg 59:7–19, 1970
20. Danielsson U, Arturson G, Wennberg L: Variations in metabolic rate in burned patients as a result of the injury and the care. Burns 5:169–173, 1978–1979
21. Warden GD, Wilmore DW, Rogers PW, Mason AD, Pruitt BA: Hypernatremic state in hypermetabolic burn patients. Arch Surg 106:420–427, 1973
22. Black S, Carter GM, Nitz AJ, Worthington JA: Oxygen consumption for lower extremity exercises in normal subjects and burn patients. Phys Ther 60: 1255–1258, 1980
23. Wilmore DW: Nutrition and metabolism following thermal injury. Clin Plast Surg 1:603–619, 1974
24. Jaeger DL: Maintenance of function of the burn patient. Phys Ther 52:627–633, 1972
25. Pruitt BA: Complications of thermal injury. Clin Plast Surg 1:667–691, 1974
26. Boswick JA: The management of fresh burns of the hand and deformities resulting from burn injuries. Clin Plast Surg 1:621–631, 1974
27. Nicosia J, Stein E, Stein J: The advantages of physiotherapy for burn patients under anesthesia. Burns 6:202–204, 1980
28. West DA, Shuck JM: Emotional problems of the severely burned patient. Surg Clin North Am 58:1189–1204, 1978
29. Edstrom LE, Robson MC: Evaluation of exercise techniques in the burn patient. Burns 4:113–117, 1978
30. Headley BJ, Robson MC, Krizek TJ: Methods of reducing environmental stress for the acute burn patient. Phys Ther 55:5–9, 1975
31. Knott M, Voss DE: Proprio-ceptive Neuromuscular Facilitation, 2nd ed. New York, Harper & Row, 1968
32. Jackson DM: Burns into joints. Burns 2:91–106, 1976
33. Achaur BM, Bartlett RH, Furnas DW, Allyn PA, Wingerson E: Internal Fixation in the management of the burned hand. Arch Surg 108:814–820, 1974
34. Wilmore DW, Aulick HL: Metabolic changes in burned patients. Surg Clin North Am 58:1178–1187, 1978
35. Whitmore JJ, Burt MM, Fowler RS, Halar E, Berni R: Bandaging the lower extremity to control swelling: figure-8 versus spiral technique. Arch Phys Med 53:487–490, 1972
36. Baur PS, Larson DL, Sloan DF, Barrett GF: An in situ procedure for the biopsy of pressure-wrapped hypertrophic scars. J Inves Dermatol 68:385–388, 1977
37. Evans EB, Larson DL, Yates S: Preservation and restoration of joint function in patients with severe burns. JAMA 204:843–848, 1968

38. Evans EB: Orthopaedic measures in the treatment of severe burns. J Bone Joint Surg 48A:643–669, 1966
39. Head MD, Helm PA: Paraffin and sustained stretching in the treatment of burn contractures. Burns 4:136–139, 1977–1978
40. Johnson CL, O'Shaughnessy EJ, Ostergren G: Burn Management. New York, Raven Press, 1981

5 | Pain and Psychological Stress Management

Irwin E. Mendelsohn

In the attempt to understand human behavior, the concept of psyche and soma, mind and body, wedded into a single holistic unit must be recognized. Issues that impact on the mind affect the body, and conversely, those affecting the body impact on the mind. Useful rehabilitation efforts must deal with both mind and body. For this reason, an indepth review of the pyschological issues involved in the management of the burn patient will follow.

In order to clarify these phenomena, certain basic psychological principles will be briefly reviewed. A basic tenet suggests that there is a reason for every emotional reaction. Psychological reactions do not occur by chance. Emotional reactions may be overt and clearly discerned, or may be hidden and not at all apparent to the subject or to the observer. This happens because of the organizational configuration of the psyche.

The mind is divided into conscious, preconscious and unconscious segments. Conscious operations take place within the full awareness of the individual. Unconscious operations occur without the individual's awareness. Preconscious issues fall between these two polarities. All thoughts, feelings, and actions reside in these segments, and there can be a constant and rapid shift from one to the other.

The human being under normal circumstances will strive to gain pleasure and avoid pain. This is true psychologically as well as physically. Psychological displeasure comes in the form of painful affect, such as anxiety, fear, anger, and guilt. In order to keep these affects buried in the unconscious mind and consequently out of the awareness, various mechanisms of defense are employed. These defenses are usually unconscious, therefore automatic, and serve to keep uncomfortable feelings out of awareness. Brief descriptions of a few of these defense mechanisms that are pertinent to our work follow.

> *Repression* implies the automatic barring from consciousness of anxiety-producing thoughts or feelings. This is the primary defense mechanism.
>
> *Regression* deals with a painful affect by moving back in time to earlier, more childlike forms of behavior. The mind attempts to create "good parents" who will nurture the individual.
>
> *Denial* is basically a refusal to accept reality. The pain-producing issue, which is externally real, does not exist for the person.
>
> *Isolation* allows the thought to emerge, but blocks the associated painful emotion.

Identification, projection, turning against oneself, reaction formation, rationalization, and *undoing* are other important defensive maneuvers used to combat anxiety. These operations are found in normal as well as pathological behavior. In pathological behavior, however, certain of these mechanisms are used excessively and inappropriately. This will lead to behavior patterns that are considered deviant.

A final principle to review in this discussion is the concept of *transference* and *countertransference.* In certain emotionally laden circumstances, people may interact with others in the same way as they dealt with significant figures from their past. Instead of visualizing the reality of the situation, images of a prior parent-child relationship emerge. The individual discards reality and operates in his fantasied past life. This leads to irrational expectations, acting out behavior, and confusion. In the patient-therapist relationship, the therapist is frequently looked upon, irrationally, as a nurturing parent. If these expectations are not met by the therapist, illogical responses by the patient can ensue. This is transference. Countertransference, however, is the reverse. Unreasonable expectations are anticipated by the therapist who, in this case, wishes the patient to be a "good child." Obviously, this too can lead to confusion, emotional upset, and acting out on the therapist's part. Because of the obvious destructive potential, an understanding of this principle is critical for the development of a truly therapeutic relationship.

Let us now examine the meaning of stress as it applies to our topic. *Stress* can be defined as any disruption of the homeostatic balance in an organism. It requires the use of adaptive mechanisms to restore that balance. This is not only limited to physiological issues, but psychological and social issues as well. In major burn trauma, all three areas are seriously affected. This stress leads to the individual's strenuous attempts to restore homeostasis in all spheres. In the process, adaptive mechanisms are severely tested, and the outcome will depend upon the success of this adaptation.

To understand the plight of the seriously burned victim, we must first look at the elements that lead to the accident. Societal statistics reveal that the majority of burn victims come from lower socioeconomic classes living in dense populations. Many burns occur in people who have an impaired or undeveloped ability to avoid danger. Such a population would include psychotics, epileptics, children, alcoholics, the elderly and/or infirm, and drug addicts.[1] McArthur and Moore found that alchoholism was the major predisposing factor in burn proneness, followed by senility, psychiatric disorder, and neurological disease.[2] The inability for self-help because of the above factors resulted in half of the fatal burns reported by Monafo.[3]

Burn trauma undoubtedly intensifies many of the individual's prior failed attempts to adjust to life, leading to further maladaptation. Obviously, these same elements will significantly create poor adjustments to the therapeutic routine, as was demonstrated in a study by Andreasen et. al.[4] The therapist must take these issues into account.

We now turn to examining what the burn victim faces from the moment of the initial catastrophe. He is abruptly confronted with an unexpected painful and life-threatening circumstance. After surviving the initial confusion of the emergency situation, he is whisked away to an unknown institution, to be cared for by strangers. His very existence is undergoing a severe test.

Initially, the patient may feel grateful for having survived the incident, but thoughts of the trauma, loss or injury to loved ones, loss of property, financial concerns, helplessness, fear, anger, and guilt soon engulf his psyche. The initial feeling of relief, because of help from the medical staff, quickly evaporates when pain becomes associated with the treatments. Later the patient has to deal with procedures in which his altered, blackened, painful body is constantly exposed, and where the therapeutic maneuvers produce further pain. Without an appetite, he is forced to take in large amounts of nutrients. Tubbings, debridement, and surgical procedures become a way of life. Isolation from friends and family, as well as virtual isolation from other patients, is a necessity, leading to further feelings of alienation. In cases where patients are attached to lifesaving medical equipment, actual sensory deprivation can occur. As the threat to survival abates, concern for future disfigurement intensifies. Throughout this entire process, the specter of pain hovers as a constant companion.

It is, therefore, easy to understand that certain psychological reactions to the above events will have to take place. Anxiety reactions, which include insomnia and emotional lability, mild depression, and fears (both realistic and unrealistic) are all part of the "normal" reactions expected after such acute trauma.[5] When these reactions become intensified and others appear, extensive interventions are required.

For clarification, it is desirable to divide the recovery process from severe burn into four overlapping phases: three during hospitalization and the fourth at home.[6] The first, or acute, phase is dominated by physiological mechanisms and emergency defenses. In the intermediate state, which usually begins after two weeks, psychological factors come strongly into play. As recovery continues, the patient enters into the third stage, where social issues influence the victim's thoughts, feelings, and behaviors. The final stage follows discharge, when the individual again has to readjust to family, job, and society. All phases interweave physiological and environmental realities, with psychological events. We will describe each of the phases below, discussing specific normal and maladaptive responses; and later, review management issues and the role of the therapeutic team in recovery.

During the first or physiological phase, the burn victim attempts to adapt to an abrupt change in status, from healthy to suddenly life-endangered. This is the time when the patient is literally fighting for his life (generally the first two to four weeks). He is undergoing anoxia, electrolyte imbalance, infection, hormonal shifts, edema, and reactions in every system complex of the body. The stress is tremendous. Psychologically, the issues are the same. In trying to cope with the clear-cut danger and fear, the victim uses primitive defenses like repression and denial to ward off reality. Reality can literally mean an extinction of life itself.

The major psychological syndromes resulting from the stresses and defenses during this first phase are delirium, insomnia, and anxiety. The delirium is based primarily on a reversible organic brain syndrome, mainly due to metabolic factors. It is characterized by confusion, disorientation, agitation or apathy, insomnia and nightmares, some intellectual impairment, and hallucinations. Neurological signs may be present. Delirium tends to be worse at night and is more common among the elderly and in patients who have a greater percent of burned area. It occurs in approximately 30 percent of adult burned patients. The clinical picture may find the patient entering a dreamlike state with little awareness of surroundings; or more commonly, the patient may demonstrate marked anxiety with emotional lability and exaggerated startle responses.[7] Commonly seen is an intensification of symptoms of delirium during impending sepsis. Cerebral edema appears to be the basic pathophysiological mechanism in delirium, as reported by Hughes and Cayaffa.[8]

Basically, the patient is attempting to psychologically minimize the impact of the injury and the threat to life it represents. Avoidance defenses are primarily used for purposes of protecting the patient from being overwhelmed by the seriousness of his situation.[9] As the organic problems come under greater control, the patient has to begin to face the reality issues more squarely. This frequently leads to feelings of depression. Thus, there is a shift from denial to depression as the individual moves from the first phase of recovery to the next.

The second, or psychological, phase finds the burn victim struggling to adjust to the full impact of his trauma. The immediate threat to life has abated, but now the patient must cope with the constant pain of his injuries and treatment. He is beginning to examine the quality of his future life. Concern over finances, family issues, career, and general losses caused by the accident come to the forefront. Worry over current and future treatment procedures, length of hospitalization, and restoration of functioning becomes prominent. Concurrently, awareness of contact with the treating personnel, family, and general surroundings is increased. Nurses, physicians, physical and occupational therapists, dietary personnel, social workers, and ward clerks are in constant interaction with the patient. The family visits become an established routine. All of these factors require further adaptation of the burn victim, who is just beginning to emerge from his sudden and severe physiological and emotional insult.

Normal psychological reactions in this phase include mild fear (related to pain of treatment), anxiety about future functioning, and mild depression resulting from grief over loss of functioning, disfigurement, and separation from loved ones. It is important to stress that these reactions are considered normal during this phase. Exaggerations, however, are pathological and generally lead to poor adaptation and serious problems in recovery. When this occurs, the syndromes of severe depression, regression, or psychosis can result. Approximately one third of adult burn patients will display pathological symptoms during their hospitalization that are severe enough to be clinically diagnosed.[5]

Depression can become a major problem in the recovery of a burn victim. Not only is the markedly saddened mood and withdrawal from contact with the outside world significant, but the generalized apathy and wish to die can actually hinder recovery. Refusal to eat, marked sleep disturbances, disinterest in exercise, and general lack of cooperation with the staff ultimately leads to decreased strength, weight loss, and contractures, which can effectively alter the prognosis. It is probable that the lack of will to live can eventuate in the actual demise of the patient. This behavior can be interpreted as an indirect form of suicide. Of course, as with any depression, the possibility of direct suicidal acting out must be considered and guarded against.

Severe regression, another psychological complication of the second stage, is characterized by a childlike, demanding behavior pattern on the part of the patient. Exaggerated dependence, the constant cry for attention, refusal to accept reality, temper tantrums, low frustration tolerance, and need for immediate personal gratification is descriptive of this syndrome. Mild regression can be helpful to the patient in that it allows him to accept a dependent role and act cooperatively with the treating personnel. Severe regression, however, is counterproductive. It creates a negative effect on the treatment team, which can have a major impact on care. Hostility, neglect, and punishment can be the staff response to severe regression. Obviously, the result of this can be extremely detrimental to the patient.

Psychosis (severe disturbance in reality testing, bizarre behavior, inappropriate emotionality, hallucinations and delusions, and feelings of persecution) is another complication of severe burn trauma. This will generally occur in an individual having a prior history of psychosis or a previous inadequate response to stress.[10] It is not uncommon to see mild forms of psychotic behavior in the form of minimal delirium during the first phase of recovery. Hallucinatory experiences and problems with reality testing can occur, but usually clear quickly once metabolic, physiological, and pharmacological issues are in balance. The reactions referred to as psychoses, however, are fixed and long lasting, possibly leading to serious consequences. The outcome of treatment plans and future adjustment are certainly adversely affected by the development of a psychotic reaction.

As previously mentioned, a good percentage of burn victims come from the impaired portion of the population. This group naturally contains a significant number of people who are actively psychotic prior to their burn. Indeed, the burn itself can be the direct result of acting out a delusion or an unsuccessful suicide attempt. Many patients will continue to demonstrate their prior psychotic behavior despite hospitalization.

An interesting observation discloses that some of these patients, despite being engaged in an active psychotic process, make a good adjustment to ward routine and treatment procedures. One can speculate that the individual attention and interest displayed by the treatment team is in great contrast to the prior neglect and disinterest occurring in their past lives. Perhaps seeing their outside world as concerned, helping, caring, and protective makes the patient more willing to join it.

During the second stage of recovery, the issue of pain attains prominence. The individual is now alert enough to sense pain. He is also contending with therapy, which includes tubbings, debridement, surgical procedures, and enforced movement of areas involved in the burn. Pain, therefore, becomes all pervasive.

As exposure to pain continues, the individual's pain threshold decreases. The previously mentioned reactions of anxiety, depression, and regression all tend to increase the subjective experience of pain. This subjective experience is also affected by prior societal and cultural factors. Some investigators feel that the psychological component of pain is a more significant factor than the physical component.[11]

Although a study by Klein and Charlton[12] indicates that patients exhibit a high frequency of well-being during therapy even in the context of painful treatments, the destructive aspects of pain on staff and patients can be clearly seen. Pain can become a medium of exchange, an almost monetary system. Pain increases the feelings of hopelessness, anxiety, and depression. The staff, having to inflict pain in treatment, has to deal with many introspective issues. Both staff and patient attempt to avoid pain-producing procedures, which can have future negative effects on treatment. Therefore, pain control is an essential management issue, which will be discussed later.

The third phase usually begins during the sixth to eighth week of hospitalization, and will be referred to as the recuperative phase. At this time, discharge from the hospital looms on the horizon. Integration of psychological factors occurs. The patient begins to deal with identity questions, looks more toward social factors, and starts considering reentry into family life and society.

Identity issues are prominent and frequently depend on the extent and anatomical location of the burn. The very integrity of self, the body, has been altered. Recognition of the changed self is difficult and anxiety-provoking. If there has been damage to the face, disfiguring scarring may make the featues unrecognizable or expressionless. If there has been burn damage to the genitalia or breasts, sexual identity disturbances will occur. The patient recognizes that burns on exposed portions of the body will be seen by others and cause reactions of fear and possibly revulsion. Posture and carriage are affected by the scarring and contractures of the healing process. Distortions of hand functions markedly impair the individual's ability to contact, touch, and express emotions. These are issues that the victim has to seriously consider during this phase of recovery.

Other issues to resolve are reentry into society and separation from the treatment team. Thoughts about career, finances, returning to home environment, and renewed sexuality are interwoven with the fear of leaving the protective burn unit atmosphere. Although most patients are anxious to return home, anxiety over future adjustments is usually present. Occasionally, a flare-up of prior maladaptation in the form of regression or depression will occur just prior to discharge or soon after.

The fourth phase of recovery can be considered the social phase. When the patient is discharged, usually back to his home environment, he has to deal with his disfigurement outside of the protective atmosphere of a burn unit. He has to return to work or school, and deal with rehabilitation attempts to return him to full function. Readjustment to family life may be difficult because of financial issues, loss of property, or loss of family members. The patient will often be left with significant disabilities leading to impairment of function. The need for frequent future hospitalizations and surgery has to be anticipated. Ongoing physical therapy can be a constant reminder of incapacitation. As a result, the pressure of adaptation is great.

In this setting, it is not surprising that patients will develop feelings of anxiety and depression. Depending on the prior psychological strength of the patient, these symptoms can be kept at a minimal level. If not, the feelings of hopelessness and guilt can intensify, fostering a full-fledged, traumatic neurosis.

The reactions of family members, friends, neighbors, and coworkers to the patient increase in importance. They frequently represent a mirror to the patient of his own recovery and self-worth. They also represent hope or hopelessness, survival or impaired survival. The patient will be acutely sensitive to the reactions he sees around him.

STAFF ISSUES

We will now more closely examine the makeup of the burn unit and the treating team. The burn unit is much like other intensive care units, but also demonstrates significant differences. As in other units, it is a place characterized by high technology, specially trained staff, team approach, and isolation. Training is mainly directed toward emergency medical and surgical care. This mix often leads to a dehumanizing situation in which the patient is viewed in a fragmented and anatomical manner. This setting also tends to put aside warm, emotional, and human contact for staff and patient alike.

There are significant differences between the burn unit and other acute care units. The sights and smells characteristic of burn injury makes for an obvious difference from other emergency care settings. Isolation of both staff and patient from the outside world is more pronounced in the burn unit primarily due to fear of infection. There is the constant issue of pain to deal with. Patients in burn centers stay longer than in other intensive care units, or indeed, any other hospital units. This results in a much more intense and prolonged patient-staff interaction, and allows for the development of considerable emotionality and acting out behavior.

The fact that the treating staff consists of a multidisciplinary team is also more apparent in the burn center. Because of the complexity of the burn injury, physicians from all specialties are involved, as well as nurses, physical and occupational therapists, dietitians, laboratory specialists, and social workers. This aggregation of people generally operates under the supervision of a burn center director, either a plastic or general surgeon. With the large number of specialists involved in the care of a patient, it is easy to see how much intrastaff friction and petty interdisciplinary jealousies can evolve. This friction worsens if the surgical leader of the team assumes a strongly authoritarian position. It is incumbent upon this leader to modulate and orchestrate the team, not dominate it. This means he has to listen to the input from various specialties and draw them into an effective, cooperative unit. It is also important for the patient to have an individual physician singled out for him as "his doctor."

In an important study by Quinley and Bernstein,[13] the adaptation of new nurses to a children's burn unit was investigated over a period of one year. The study is applicable to other personnel, such as physical therapists and occupational therapists, who become intensely involved with burn patient care. At first, the beginning nurses would express a great deal of enthusiasm about their future work. Their image was one of a "super nurse" with highly developed technical skills. They envisioned themselves as counselors, consultants, and psychotherapists, and did not think that their own feelings would become a serious (core) problem. The nurses approached the negative reactions concerning work in the burn unit, mainly expressed by fellow professionals, by accepting it as a personal challenge. They later had a great deal of difficulty in discussing their unique problems with these peers because of a basic lack of understanding. The initial expectation of receiving admiration from others for their work, of not being upset by the emotionally laden experiences they encountered, and of being accepted as loveable authority figures by their patients did not materialize.

When the nurse had to engage in pain-producing treatments, feelings of anxiety and professional incompetence arose. They became exhausted by these feelings, which were stimulated during the repetitive treatments, and frustrated at not being able to alter the patients' reactions to their pain-producing activity. They responded to the angry outbursts from the patients by becoming angry themselves. This, in turn, was followed by feelings of guilt and shame. Maintaining a distance from the patient then became a protective mechanism. To justify their behavior, the nurses created doubts about the reality of the patient's pain. Was the patient faking it, or was it real?

At this point, the nurses became concerned over the quality of life the deformed patients would subsequently lead. They overidentified with their patients, feeling similar resentment and humiliation concerning current and future disfigurement. This resulted in overpraising and lack of objectivity.

As time went on, a more realistic picture of limited goals emerged. The rescue fantasy finally had to be abandoned. There developed a growing acceptance that perfectionistic and idealized goals were unrealistic. This led to greater flexibility in dealing with patients and family. Temporary states of depression, anxiety, and hostility amongst the staff were accepted and understood. Group feelings emerged as they became veterans in their work. The mechanisms of denial and emotional distancing became more subtle and were more constructively used. Causing pain created much sympathy and empathy without overwhelming feelings of guilt and anxiety. The nurses finally felt gratification from their important, realistic contributions.

As we can visualize, similar factors apply to any member of the treatment team who has close patient contact. The setting of realistic goals and achieving gratification from limited results is important. Understanding the use of personal defenses in dealing with the rigors of burn therapy significantly adds to the ability of the therapist to treat such patients.

In this light, let us review the concepts of transference and countertransference mentioned earlier. From the patient's standpoint, they are relatively helpless in caring for themselves and are in virtually constant pain. The staff is seen as capable of nurturing them and restoring their health. It is a situation where the parental role is thrust upon the healers. When this occurs, it is usually accompanied by unrealistic expectations of the staff. Consequently, hostility, demanding regressive behavior, and depression quickly follow.

The staff, on the other hand, may assume a parental role (countertransference) and make demands on the patient to become the good, compliant child. When patients do not respond in this way, acting out by staff members in the form of rejection, anger, punishment, and infantalizing will take place. One can easily see that neither situation is conducive to optimum care. Spillover from these situations to other family members occurs and can also lead to inadequate management. In a study concerning adaptation of patients, the single most important factor in sustaining hope and morale was visitations by the spouse or close family members. If relationships with these visiting people become significantly impaired because of transferential issues, the patient will again become the victim.

One of the most difficult matters the staff has to deal with is death and dying. It will often evoke the strongest psychological reactions of the treatment process. This is particularly true when the staff is confronted with a dying patient who can be closely identified with. Children, young adults, or patients having similar character-istics to staff members and who are close to death create group grief reactions. The longer the patient has been on the unit, the more severe are the reactions.

The dying patient goes through the stages, as described by Kubler-Ross, of denial, anger, bargaining, depression, and finally acceptance.[15] These stages set up staff reactions that lead to rejection, anger, detachment, and finally guilt. Self-reproach, accusations, and strong feelings of failure will often follow. Confidence in one's self and fellow team members can be destroyed by these feelings, and staff morale can deteriorate quickly. Ventilation of thoughts and feelings at a time like this is most important, particularly if done in a group setting. The sense of sharing frustrations, feelings of inadequacy, and guilt with other team members is very ther-apeutic.

Aside from death, daily team pressures include viewing mutilations and disfig-urement, inflicting pain, dealing with emergency situations, and managing feelings associated with the patient's sexual exposure. In this setting, stoicism amongst the staff, as well as within the patient, is encouraged. The individual staff member or patient that can stand up to the rigors of treatment is looked upon with respect. Stoicism, however, can be counterproductive and will often prevent the necessary ventilation of thoughts and feelings, leading to greater stress in the individuals in-volved.

The smooth running of the team requires frequent communication and contact among its members. Regular team meetings facilitate this process. It not only pro-vides for a sharing of information and treatment planning, but also allows for expres-sion of emotions, which is necessary for morale.

We must remain cognizant of the fact that the burn unit is part of a greater hospital structure. Hospital policies and attitudes have a strong impact on the unit. Issues such as staffing, hours, pay, and recognition of unique problems of the unit are very important to adequate functioning. In this light, administrative support is critical: it will quickly reflect down to the level of direct patient care. The support and cooperation of the ancillary services such as other medical and psychological specialties, nursing, physical therapy, occupational therapy, rehabilitation medicine, dietary, and social services must be provided. It is very often the team member from an ancillary service that offers important feedback to the medical members of the team. For example, the physical therapist and occupational therapist, because of their prolonged contact with the patient, can be important listening posts during the treatment sessions. Patients will often feel more comfortable discussing matters of inner concern with the nonphysician team members. Information gathered here and shared with the rest of the staff is invaluable.

MANAGEMENT

In the discussion of management, we will be primarily concerned with the psychological aspects of patient care. We have described earlier the desperate position that patient and family abruptly find themselves in following a major burn. We have also delineated the four stages found in recovery from this injury. We now turn to a discussion of some general treatment measures, followed by a review of specific, phase-related techniques.

The single most important psychological issue in the care of the patient is warm human contact. This runs through the entire spectrum of the treatment process. The need for compassion, empathy, guidance, interest, and support is paramount, and can only be provided by another caring human being. Early, when treatment attention is focused on the physiological concern, medical attention given with empathy fulfills that requirement. Later, as the patient progresses into other phases of recovery, care by other team members provided in this same manner will continue to fulfill that need. This empathy has the quality of nurturing and can be likened to maternal caring. It provides the individual with the necessary security during the time of severe stress. One should not use preoccupation with technical matters as an excuse to forget about the importance of empathy.

As recovery progresses, the nurturing aspect of care should begin to ease. As with the child who is growing up, more and more is expected from the patient. Growth and independence should be encouraged, but only at the pace that is suitable for the individual. If accomplished, overdependency and invalidism are prevented, and the momentum for rehabilitation is established. The patient can look forward to a maximal recovery.

Qualities of compassion and empathy cannot be taught. However, through staff interaction and exploration of shared experiences, these qualities can be enhanced. Introspection for this purpose should become part of every serious training program. Our patients require it.

Another critical element in the general psychological management of the patient is the provision of adequate and clear information concerning the damage, treatment, and prognosis. Nothing promotes anxiety more rapidly than not knowing the what, how, and why of an illness and treatment. When a patient is appropriately informed about these matters, it allows him to assume some control over the problem. This sense of control can be very reassuring.

The issue of communication between patient and therapist is a complex matter. It involves psychological factors in both therapist and patient. The therapist, through his or her own anxiety, may remain silent and not address the issues with the patient at all. Occasionally, in attempts to explain therapy, complicated physiological or medical terminology may be used, confusing the patient but allowing the therapist to feel that communication has taken place. Occasionally, therapists hide behind the idea that the patient could not understand the complexities involved; therefore, not giving him information is somehow protective. This is an erroneous conclusion. A simple, clear, and concise explanation given at the comprehension level of the patient will usually be understood and appreciated.

There are times, however, when the explanation will not be understood. This will occur when the patient is not emotionally ready to hear what is being said.[16] The patient using the defense mechanism of denial to control the overwhelming feelings of anxiety will often block out information. The communication will only be integrated when the patient is finally able to accept it emotionally. When blocking occurs, as angry confrontation between patient and therapist over what was, or was not, said will often ensue. To avoid this situation, frequent repetition may be required. This could be accompanied by asking the patient questions in order to see what level of comprehension was attained.

Honesty in dealing with patients is very important. One should not be afraid to say, "I don't know," if one doesn't know. The patient will accept the lack of knowledge much more readily than he would dishonesty. Honesty enhances rapport and trust, both major factors in the therapeutic process. In the climate of trust, the patient will tolerate virtually any procedure asked of him. When trust is lacking, an uncooperative patient is the result.

A word should be mentioned about bedside rounds, which is looked upon by staff as routine daily work. The patient, however, sees it as an important time to learn about his treatment, prognosis, and so on. It is also a time to register complaints, concerns, and requests. Unfortunately for the patient however, this rarely takes place. He is generally confronted with a group of specialists talking in a "foreign" language amongst themselves, but obviously about him. Little or no time is spent either talking to or listening to the patient himself. He is often left with many unanswered questions, and perhaps a perfunctory "You're doing well" or "We are planning a debridement later today." One can see how anxiety can be intensified by such an event.

Rounds should include the patient. Instead of making him an object, he should be made a participant. This is not to say that differences over therapeutic approaches should include the patient's opinion. Those discussions should take place away from the bedside. The final resolution of these issues should be presented to the patient, and time given to him for a response. Doing this allows the patient to feel a greater control over what is happening to him. Control, however limited, is important to the patient. Actual choice by the patient of the type and intensity of treatment is allowed in some burn centers. In a report from the University of Southern California,[17] the choice of aggressive care versus normal, comforting care is made by the patient in severe burn situations. This has not changed mortality statistics, but has increased the contact and empathy of the treating team.

The patient should be allowed as much self-care as is possible, depending upon his stage of recovery. Participation in dressing changes, decision-making when confronted with equal alternatives, and personal hygiene must be encouraged. It gives the individual a sense of control, which will go a long way in the prevention of overdependency.

In discussing the general psychological aspects involved in patient care, one should not forget that the burn unit is also a social unit for the patient. Aside from obvious involvement with the staff, there is an important network established with other patients. At first, when the patient is obtunded, isolated, and connected to various pieces of "hardware," social aspects are minimal and limited to staff interaction. As the patient progresses to the point of ambulation, more and more contact is made with the other patients. The sharing of experiences, both pre and postburn can assume the level of a local support system. Feelings toward various staff members can be ventilated in this informal way. Discussions over various treatments undergone lead to a certain camaraderie.

Most patients are aware of all the ward events, including emergencies and deaths. These matters directly affect morale and should be dealt with rapidly by the treating staff. The anxiety relating to such events as "Joe over there died last night, what about me?" must be relieved as soon as possible.

Occasionally this ward support system is enhanced by the return of a former patient. This veteran group can be very helpful in seeing current patients through their individual difficulties. Patients are often more open with others who have had similar experiences, and this sharing can be most therapeutic. The veteran group also provides living examples of recovery and, therefore, hope. With a small amount of training, these former patients can become useful adjunctive therapists. Formal burn recovery groups have been formed in various centers around the country for this purpose.

PAIN MANAGEMENT

As stated earlier, the issues of pain and its ramifications assume great importance in the treatment of the burn patient. Pain is the signal to the individual that something is terribly awry. As pain intensity increases, the perception of danger in the form of threat to life emerges. This is accompanied by great anxiety, which in turn increases pain perception.

It is, therefore, clear that basic management techniques should include listening carefully to the patient. Allow the individual to freely and fully express his concerns. *This willingness to listen signifies staff interest and empathy, two vital factors in establishing rapport.*

After allowing ventilation of emotions to take place, *reassurance* should be the next step. An honest appraisal of what might be expected in the future concerning pain and treatment should be stated. Doing this enhances the position of the therapist as being a knowledgeable, honest person, who is in control of the treatment program. Feelings of trust are developed. The cornerstones of a good therapeutic program are rapport and trust.

More specific management techniques used for pain control include analgesic medication, anesthesia, hypnosis, biofeedback, transcutaneous electrical stimulation, and behavioral modification. A more-detailed discussion of each of these techniques will follow.

Although there is uniform agreement that pain control is most desirable, the use of analgesic agents for this purpose is controversial. Most people place pain control high on the list in importance; yet many feel that analgesic agents currently in use are ineffective in preventing perception of pain in burns. In addition, these agents, such as morphine, demerol, and so on, have a high addiction potential, particularly when used over a long period of time. Central nervous system depression, possibly interfering with an already compromised respiratory and circulatory physiology, is also of major concern. These agents, by causing unwanted sedation, retard physical movement, which increases muscle wasting and joint stiffness, making later rehabilitation efforts more difficult. In addition, they also cause gastrointestinal hypomobility and decreased appetite at a time when the patient's enteral needs may be two to three times the norm.

Despite the above issues, the judicious use of analgesic agents is recommended by most physicians. Many feel addiction will take place in only those patients who are addiction-prone. Titrating doses carefully and monitoring the patients closely can make for a successful outcome. Since a large component of pain perception is anxiety, the use of minor tranquilizers, such as diazepam may be an important adjunct for treatment. The process of giving the patient medication also communicates the idea of "we care about you" which has its own obvious importance.

Anesthesia is probably underutilized, particularly during dressing changes. A major reason for this is the difficulty in obtaining full-time anesthesia coverage in a burn center. General anesthesias and agents like ketamine have been used in areas where such coverage was obtainable.[18] In a most interesting paper published by Thal et al. in 1979, workers at the University of Texas used self-administered nitrous oxide for relief of pain during emergencies, including burns.[19] They report 93 percent of patients achieved total or partial relief of pain, and that the procedure was safe and well-tolerated. Further work in this area is needed.

Hypnosis is another modality employed in burn patient management, and has been used since approximately 1955. The technique provides generalized relaxation as well as direct blocking of pain during procedures. In a study by Wakeman and Kaplan, patients treated with hypnosis required less analgesia, enhanced their ego strengths, and possibly improved their appetites.[20]

The use of relaxation techniques and hypnosis can be especially helpful to the physiotherapist. With the resulting increased muscle relaxation and decreased pain perception, greater exercise and movement demands can be placed on the patient. There is also a greater willingness by the patient to perform tasks that before would have been considered impossible.

In certain burns where chronic pain in an area is the outcome, the use of biofeedback should be considered. In one study, pain was reduced and possible nerve regeneration enhanced with this technique.[21]

The use of transcutaneous electrical stimulation (TENS) for pain relief must also be considered. It has been used effectively in various burn centers, and this approach again warrants further investigation.

Behavioral modification can be a very useful modality, particularly in the management of pain in children or regressed adults. The reinforcement given by way of reward for lack of negative response to pain proved to be a successful management technique. A study by Varni et al. showed the effectiveness of this technique during the physical therapy of a three-year-old girl.[22]

Other behavioral techniques such as desensitization, modelling, operant conditioning, and environmental manipulation have also been used successfully. The importance of pain management cannot be overemphasized. Any safe and effective method should be used.

PSYCHOLOGICAL MANAGEMENT DURING THE FOUR PHASES

A discussion of specific treatment techniques that are primarily useful in each phase of recovery will follow. Case reports will be given as examples.

During stage one, the patient is reacting mainly to his physiological stresses. Following an initial calm, both the body and mind begin to cope with the pressure of anoxia, acidosis, fluid depletion, and so on. This can lead to the impairments described earlier. If the stress is severe enough, delerium will be the result.

The initial step in the treatment of delerium is to determine the underlying physiological causes and correct them where possible. While this search proceeds, reduction and prevention of excessive anxiety and helplessness is important.[23] This can be accomplished by reassurance ("you'll be all right"), relaxation ("try to relax"), passivity encouragement ("we'll take care of you"), gentle encouragement ("try to put up with it"), and self-participation ("give us a hand"). Touching the patient is important, especially when verbal communication is not possible. Being in close physical proximity with the seriously burned individual is also helpful in countering fears of abandonment.

Sensory input, in general, is needed to combat the effects of delerium. Clocks, TV, radios, and personnel should give constant orientation input. Unconditional support must be available. The patient and family should be reassured that the problem is self-limited and not a result of going crazy. Information relating to the actual accident should be provided, but only to the point where the patient can accept it. The patient himself must be the guide.

In many cases, control of agitation and psychotic symptoms must include the use of neuroleptic medications.[24] These major tranquilizers (phenothiazines, haloperidol, etc.) can be most effective in controlling agitation, delusional thinking, and hallucinations. In addition, the use of any modality that inhibits physical movement should be limited. Immobilization does contribute to delerium as well as joint stiffness and wound contracture.

Case History #1: Mr. B, a 34-year-old married man with two children, worked as a glass installer for many years. He suffered a severe electrical burn during an attempt to extricate a fellow worker from a truck that had a high voltage wire lying on the chassis. The electrical charge arced from one hand to the other, causing damage to both. Internal injuries were not initially apparent, but were anticipated. At the time of the accident, the patient was certain he was dying. Before losing consciousness he felt as if he were being propelled, frighteningly, through a long, dark tunnel. Then he found himself in a beautiful setting, only again to return to the feared tunnel.

After making a reasonably good adjustment to the ward routine and to the ongoing medical ministrations, he began complaining of increasing insomnia. He could not sleep when darkness came. Increasing agitation and confusion followed. Neurological investigation did not reveal any positive findings. It soon became clear that he was unable to sleep because of recurring dreams and daytime thoughts of going through the feared tunnel again. This increased his agitation considerably. The tunnel became a frightening, virtually hallucinatory event and filled all of his waking hours. Continued medical investigation did not reveal any physiological findings to explain the symptomatology.

The patient was reassured that his visions would decrease in frequency and intensity as time went on. He was started on Thorazine. At night he was allowed to leave his bed, sit at the nurses' station, and converse with the staff. After approximately one to two weeks, there was a significant decrease in symptoms. He was better able to verbalize more about the accident and the subsequent feelings of panic associated with going through the tunnel. The Thorazine was discontinued, and the patient made an uneventful psychological recovery.

Another brief example demonstrates how delerium could be easily missed by the staff.

Case History #2: A middle-aged man was admitted to the burn center with approximately 30 percent second- and third-degree burns following a gasoline explosion. He appeared to be making an uncomplicated recovery. No aberrant behavior was seen by the treating personnel, and the patient did not report having any unusual problems. In casual conversation with the unit psychiatrist about one month after admission, the patient said, "Doc., I would like to tell you about this funny experience I had during the first week I was here. I used to watch television all day long because there was nothing else to do. But at night, when the lights were out, I kept seeing a little man sitting on top of the television set, looking at me. I was afraid to tell anyone about this because they would think I'm nuts. But after a few weeks, it went away." The patient was finally able to admit to visual hallucinations only when the visions left. He was never treated with major tranquilizers and was eventually discharged. One can wonder how often the acute brain syndrome occurs unnoticed in our patient population.

Anxiety and pain, as discussed earlier, are recurring and dominant themes during the second stage of recovery. In treating mild to moderate anxiety, all the general approaches mentioned before are important. In addition, the judicious use of minor tranquilizers (Valium, Tranxene) can be extremely helpful. Should symptomatology intensify, the syndromes of regression, depression, or psychosis can result. In these situations, psychiatric intervention is indicated.

In the regressed patient, the individual is trying to cope by presenting himself in a childlike manner. This often generates much staff anger.[16] In dealing with this situation, the staff should encourage whatever appropriate adult behavior is present by remaining firm and consistent in setting limits. Openly telling the patient about how his regressive attitude directly causes anger can help create an improved atmosphere. As mentioned earlier, behavior modification can be useful. Reward for desirable behavior can work where other techniques fail. Often regression cannot be adequately dealt with, and the patient's progress will be impaired. Should an individual staff member find himself unable to cope with a specific regressed patient, contact between these two should be limited if possible.

Case History #3:   A 59-year-old white male factory supervisor was admitted with 36 percent third-degree burns on his lower extremities following a gasoline fire. His psychological history indicated that he generally operated in a rather authoritarian manner before the accident. He was used to giving orders and also used to having people obey them. This was especially true of his wife and family.

His hospital stay was characterized by an initial depression, quickly followed by apathy and lack of motivation. He became childlike and demanding, and frequently resisted attempts to get him to follow ward routine. This behavior was particularly manifested during physiotherapy attempts and when his wife visited. He would refuse to follow instructions and often coerced his wife to perform tasks that were part of his therapy. He consistently asked for assistance and usually needed standby supervision. If refused, he became petulant.

During his long stay, much time was spent constantly reassuring and encouraging him. Limits were set by not acquiescing to his constant demands. Reward in the form of positive reinforcement and encouragement was given. His wife was included in this limit-setting approach. Finally, albeit slowly, he was able to ambulate. This encouraged him to make more progress until he was finally discharged.

Depression is a frequent condition seen in this second stage. Patients will often grieve inwardly, preventing others from being aware of their depression; but, if encouraged to talk, depressive feelings could be expressed, substantially minimizing the impact. Permission to openly cry can also be very therapeutic. Reassurance that depression often follows this kind of injury and that it is a self-limiting problem for most is helpful.

It is important to encourage visitation by family and friends as soon as possible. This contact reinforces the idea that the patient is not alone and not forgotten. Another useful technique in the prevention of depression is the promotion of physical activity, especially in helping other patients. This acts to increase self-esteem.

In certain circumstances, depression is severe and can lead to covert suicidal behavior (e.g., not eating or not cooperating with the therapeutic regimen) or overt suicidal behavior. It may become necessary to use antidepressant medication (Imipramine, Amitryptaline) when the patient is physically able to tolerate it. Although these drugs are generally effective, the fact that they can take at least two to three weeks before they act places great limitations on their usefullness. There is hope that more rapid onset medications will become available in the near future.

Case History #4:   A 54-year-old woman was admitted to the burn center following a natural gas explosion that caused 32 percent second- and third-degree burns primarily of her back. She had a stormy course that consisted of septic shock on two occasions. Because of a prior neurological condition, bladder retention was present. This made her vulnerable to repeated urinary tract infections.

During much of the time, her general psychological state was one of depression. She spoke haltingly, cried frequently, and expressed great concern over future functioning. Psychiatric consultation determined that she was suffering from a reactive depression that was intensified by her precarious and unstable medical condition.

Supportive psychotherapy was instituted. Antidepressant medication was not used because of her poor metabolic state. The use of analgesics for pain relief was strongly recommended, as was the use of minor tranquilizers. This patient had a very involved and interested family; therefore, visitation was encouraged. Although requiring repeated surgical procedures, she became more responsive to the staff. Her pessimism lifted and interaction with her family improved. Ten to twelve weeks following surgery, physical therapy was intensified and gradual ambulation was started. This was accompanied by a significant improvement in mood. She was discharged with minimal depressive signs.

Case History #5:   An attractive 21-year-old divorced mother accidentally set fire to her dress, causing second- and third-degree burns of her upper chest and neck. A few areas of first-degree burns were present on her face. Shortly following admission, the patient expressed great concern over her burns and her future appearance. As time progressed, it became evident that her current fiance was not visiting her. This intensified her concern about her appearance. She became moderately depressed, characterized by withdrawal from interaction with the staff, frequent crying episodes, sad moods, and diminished appetite. Brief psychotherapy was instituted.

It was learned that her concern with her appearance related primarily to the burns on the upper part of her breasts. This made her feel that eventually she would become sexually unattractive. She felt that her fiance's lack of visitation was an indication of this. The patient was also preoccupied with thoughts of losing her job, and worried over the care of her infant son. The ventilation of these concerns seemed to help her mood. Gradually, healing became evident. Following considerable staff encouragement, her fiance started regular visits. She became more secure with her eventual appearance, and there were no signs of depression by the time she was discharged.

Case History #6:   A middle-aged mother of two was admitted to the burn center with self-inflicted third-degree burns of the breast and upper abdomen. This incident occurred during her hospitalization for depression in a local psychiatric institution.

There was a history of severe depression for approximately six months prior to the current psychiatric hospitalization. Her depression was characterized by isolation, psychomotor retardation, and much somatic preoccupation. She felt that she was going blind despite the reassurance from several ophthalmologists.

Following the burn, her hospital course was characterized by isolation from fellow patients and staff, negativism, and somatic preoccupation (she felt her skin would be permanently stained by the medications). She ate poorly and would not allow certain treatments to be given. The patient was strongly encourage to take antidepressant medication, but she refused. Her husband supported her decision.

Despite her poor psychological state, her burns eventually healed and she neared discharge. The continued depth of the depression was reviewed with the patient and her husband. A recommendation that she remain hospitalized for psychiatric treatment was made. Both patient and her husband denied the severity of the depression and requested discharge. Approximately one week after the discharge, the patient became so retarded and negativistic that psychiatric hospitalization was finally accepted.

Psychosis is another problem that can emerge during this second stage. A number of patients admitted to the burn unit have had prior psychiatric histories of psychoses. Occasionally, the burn itself may be the result of the acting out of psychotic behavior. Management of psychotic behavior in these instances is critical to treatment.

In frank delusional behavior, phenothiazines or other major tranquilizers become important. These medications are very effective in controlling hallucinations and delusions and the rage that often underlies them. The medication, however, is not a substitute for empathic involvement by the staff. The attention, warmth, and encouragement given by concerned people in the hospital may be the first time somebody has displayed such feelings toward these patients. Frequently, the patient responds faster to this involvement than to the major tranquilizers.

When delusions are present, the patient should be allowed to express his or her thoughts. Feelings that accompany the delusional thoughts should be expressed as well. The staff members should firmly, but not argumentatively or condescendingly, deny the delusions. Reality should be presented as it exists. This will help the patient to focus more easily on the facts, and this, in itself, can be very reassuring.

It is also important to remember that many of these patients come from disturbed family situations. Dealing with family members, consequently, may require the same approach that one uses when dealing with the disturbed patient. Future medical and physical therapy planning should take this into consideration.

Case History #7:   A psychologically depressed 50-year-old married father was admitted with second-and third-degree burns of the hands, arm, chest, and neck following a suicide attempt by self-immolation. He had been despondent for the piror six months following the death of his mother and the loss of his job as a highly successful major executive in a large corporation. During this time, he had received psychiatric help and had been placed on Elavil, which he had not been able to tolerate. His ruminations and despondency deepened and finally culminated in the suicidal act. He had a past history of occasional depressive incidents for approximately fifteen years prior to his admission.

When first seen, he appeared guilt-ridden and embarrassed over what he had done. Depressive ruminations filled his thoughts and a suicidal potential remained. Flat affect and retarded activity was evident. Some cognitive dysfunction was also apparent. He denied delusions or hallucinations. A diagnosis of depression with possible underlying psychosis was made. As time went on, his symptoms remained static. As soon as his medical condition stabilized, the patient was placed on antidepressant medication (Norpramin 50 mg., three times a day).

After two weeks, his depression began to lift. He became more cooperative with the staff and assisted them in his care. He allowed visitation after initially refusing to see his wife and children. Soon, however, he became quiet, moved about restlessly, and began mumbling to himself. He appeared actively delusional and reported hallucinations. The patient was convinced that he went home every night, only to return to the hospital for treatment during the day. When his roommate was on the phone, he felt certain that the call was about him, and he therefore would join in the conversation. At one point, he thought that it was his wedding day, claiming to have seen one of the nurses wearing a bridal gown. Concern arose that an organic process, such as sepsis, was triggering this reaction.

A thorough medical search for an organic causality was unproductive. Although antidepressants have been known to cause psychotic behavior, this did not seem to be the case here. The impression was that a basic psychotic process existed and that the depression masked the psychosis. Once the depression was lifted, this psychotic process emerged.

The dose of antidepressant medication was lowered and the patient was placed on Stelcazine, 2 mg., a major tranquilizer. Symptoms were finally controlled by this maneuver and recovery proceeded.

Case History #8: A 16-year-old attractive white female was admitted with 65 percent third-degree burns to the chest, abdomen, arms, and face, following an attempt at self-immolation, which eventually caused her house to burn down. She had been a pretty, popular young lady with an ostensibly good life adjustment until her parents decided to divorce. Her mother, who had a long past psychiatric history, went to live out of state. Her father remarried a young woman not much older than the patient herself.

For the year prior to the burn incident, the patient had become more and more withdrawn. She hardly engaged socially and spent much of the time alone in her room. As time progressed, she developed marked religious preoccupation. All of her outside activities were spent in church. Later, a full-blown phobia ensued, preventing the patient from attending school. Life became intolerable, and the patient decided to kill herself. The triggering incident occurred when her stepmother, who had left her father for one week, was about to return home after a reconciliation.

Following admission, the patient continued to have delusions and hallucinations with mainly religious themes. In the past, she had been overwhelmed by guilt, feeling herself to be evil and the cause of her parent's problems. This continued to trouble her during the hospitalization. Treatment was limited to supportive psychotherapy because of the severity of her injury. This seemed to help relieve some of the guilt she felt about herself. Unfortunately, the patient developed sepsis. Attempts at resuscitation failed, and she died in her 20th hospital day.

The third phase of recovery is one of recuperation and rehabilitation. Management is directed towards preparing the patient for life outside of the hospital. The wounds are quite healed, and now function becomes the primary concern. The physiotherapist plays an even more prominent role at this time. The importance of physical rehabilitation need not be reviewed here, but the psychological impact that the therapist has on patients should not be overlooked. The patient and physiotherapist spend many hours together, and at this time, these sessions may be the patient's major social outlet. This contact affords a great opportunity for informal supportive psychotherapy to take place. The sensitive therapist knows that the patient must be prepared to deal with future dysfunction and deformity. He must be ready to leave the supportive confines of the hospital environment. He must face the difficulty in reentering the social scene. He must deal with cosmetic problems and their impact on family members and society in general.

In all of this, the empathy, trust, and rapport that was built during the other phases of recovery should provide the atmosphere for a therapeutic alliance. Allowing the patient to ventilate in a supportive milieu is extremely helpful.

Role playing is another technique that can actively prepare the patient to deal with future confrontations. By doing this, the therapist becomes a mirror of society, allowing the patient to experiment with reactions and responses. At this phase, the family should be more actively brought into future planning. Social Service, having had continuous family contacts throughout hospitalization, is in a particularly important position for effecting a smooth transition from hospital to home.

It should be recognized that a patient's optimistic view of leaving the hospital may not be a good indicator of future adjustment. It is mainly the individual's preburn personality and life adjustment abilities that will dictate how well the patient will fare. To a lesser degree, the amount of disfigurement and deformity will also be important determinants.[25]

Formal psychotherapy should be continued in those patients suffering a continued traumatic neurosis, phobia, depression, psychosis, or difficulty in dealing with deformity and dysfunction. Preparation for continuing therapy on the outside should be made during this phase; however, there remains a consistently large dropout rate in posthospitalization patients.

The major purpose of therapeutic endeavors during the stage of recovery is to reestablish the patient's identity on realistic grounds. It is this identity that must be positive enough to carry over to his home environment, so that maximal adjustment can be made.

The fourth phase of recovery, the return home, is basically a continuation of recuperation and rehabilitation phases. The difference is that now the patient must face the outside world alone, unprotected by the sympathetic hospital personnel. Factors such as the amount, type, and location of deformity, maturity of the individual, narcissism, age, sex (there is a greater emphasis on female attractiveness), family, and social support strongly influence the adaptive results.

Management should be directed toward supporting the development of a new identity. The patient, in his attempt to integrate this, has various mechanisms at his disposal.

The process of progressive desensitization begins as soon as the patient arrives home. As time goes on, there is less reaction to the individual's outward deformity. In addition, frequent reassurance about the worthiness of the individual is provided by friends and family. Confidence is slowly increased. For many, this process will go on for at least a year; for others, a lifetime.

Patients will also use rationalization and religiosity to readapt. The feeling that the ordeal "made me a better person," or "I was spared to do better things with my life" can spur an individual to work hard toward higher goals. The increased appreciation of a spouse or other family members is another frequent outcome. All of this occurs because life has become a precious gift.

Dissociation and reworking are other mechanisms operating in this phase. Some people suffer a complete loss of memory for events surrounding the trauma. Others will remember in piecemeal fashion, allowing the slow reworking of the events. This remembering, if accompanied by ventilation, decreases the painful effect associated with the trauma.

Continuing support should be provided by the treatment team in the outpatient setting. Ventilation should be encouraged. The goal of mastery and control, leading to a heightened self-esteem and positive individual identity, can then result. In a study by Mlott et al., no significant emotional or intellectual deterioration took place one year after hospitalization in adults, excluding premorbid problems.[26] Thus, some sense of optimism can be allowed.

Sadly, however, many patients do not make an adequate adjustment outside of the hospital. There is a large dropout rate from medical treatment, indicating serious flaws in our therapeutic attempts.[27] The development of traumatic neurosis and phobic neurosis leading to severe complications in living style are, unfortunately, not unusual. The spectre of future suicide can be a constant concern to families, friends, and therapists. Anecdotal reports appear to indicate a higher suicide rate in this group as compared with the normal population. Drug addiction, either preburn or iatrogenically induced, is also higher in this group. *Social death*, a term used by MacGregor to describe social withdrawal, can, unfortunately, be a frequent outcome.[28]

The treatment of children adds another dimension to this complex problem, as the child is not an isolated individual. Parents and family become crucial in the management of the child through all phases of recovery. The parents must be included in the treatment plans from the start. Since figures for disturbed behavior in children postburn vary from 20 percent to 80 percent, parents must be taught to expect behavior that would not normally have been anticipated before the burn. They have to be prepared for aggressive acting out and withdrawal, and should be given management advice and outlets.[29]

Parents must learn nursing and physical therapeutic techniques. These should be performed before discharge and under the supervision of the therapist and a nurse. Because of significant problems amongst disfigured children attempting social reentry, as reported by Molinaro, parents should be prepared to help their child cope with peer rejection.[30] A treatment manual and phone access to the staff following discharge can be very reassuring and comforting in times of stress.

A special word should be mentioned about family support groups. Bringing together family members with staff at regular meetings can be a most productive therapeutic experience.[31] The sharing of emotions, expressions of fear and guilt, discussion of treatment approaches and plans, and general feeling of emotional support is often invaluable. Although rarely provided, the need for such groups continues beyond discharge. Families have to learn to be both supporting and appropriately demanding of the patient. Occasionally, reorganization of family roles becomes necessary. Family groups are perfectly designed to handle such problems. Undoubtedly, more efforts to form such groups should be made in the future.

Case History #9:   A 28-year-old man was admitted to the burn center with 20 percent third-degree electrical burns of his right arm and leg. He was employed as a TV installer and accidentally touched a live wire. At the time of the injury, he was living with two siblings and his mother, who had divorced his father a number of years earlier. The patient was very active in outdoor sports and carpentry. He was engaged to a young woman whom he was planning to marry in the near future.

On admission, the patient expressed many concerns about survival and what his future would be like. These feelings became intensified when his lower right arm and hand became cold and cyanotic. Amputation of the extremity became necessary. After a discussion of the anticipated procedure, the patient became markedly depressed. Much time was spent crying, and he significantly withdrew from contact with the staff. Psychiatric consultation was obtained. Discussions centered on the feelings related to the forthcoming amputation. His depression was obvious. No antidepressant medication was prescribed, but supportive psychotherapy was instituted. A careful explanation of the use of prostheses by the physical therapy and rehabilitation staff was given.

Following surgery, the depression intensified. He talked of wearing a hook, which indicated how negative he felt about his future. Staff conferences with the psychiatrist were aimed at developing an improved educational and supportive program for the patient. Repetitive discussions on the types of prostheses and their functioning were held. He was encouraged to ventilate his feelings and talk about his depressive thoughts. Outward display of his emotional state was not prohibited.

Approximately ten days after his surgery, the patient's spirits began to lift, despite the fact that his wedding day would have been that weekend. Fortunately, his fiancée had very warm and loving feelings for the patient. She, and the other members of his family, including the divorced father, visited constantly. The staff had frequent contact with all of them and was therefore in an excellent position to build rapport and act in a fully supportive role.

The patient was soon ambulating and began his preprostheses work. The depression faded fairly dramatically at this point. Contact with vocational rehabilitation services was established through Social Service, and future careers were discussed.

After one more month at the burn center, he was transferred to the rehabilitation ward, where he was fitted with his prosthesis. He was eventually discharged and continued his therapy in the outpatient department. Continued support to family and patient was given by the staff during his visits to the burn outpatient clinic, as well as in the rehabilitation center where he continued his physical therapy. He later married his fiancée and currently has one child. In preparation for a new career, he attends school. His interest in outdoor activities remains. There are no significant negative psychological sequelae noted at this time.

In summary, there are three major psychological tasks that we must help our patients perform both during hospitalization and after discharge.

1. Mobilization of hope
2. The restoration of self-esteem
3. The rebuilding of interpersonal relationships

If we can accomplish these tasks, we will have achieved the goal of therapy. Psyche and soma will be reunited for the purpose of serving an effective, self-reliant, and contented individual.

REFERENCES

1. Sanders, R: The burnt patient: a general view. Br Med J 3(5928): 460–463, 1974
2. MacArthur JD, Moore FD: Epidemiology of burns. J AMC Med Assoc 231:259, 1975
3. Monafo WW: The Treatment of Burns: Principles and Practice. St. Louis, Green, 1971
4. Andreasen NJC, Noyes R, Hartford CE: Factors influencing adjustment of burn patients during hospitalization. Psychoso Med 34:6, 1972

5. Andreasen NJC: Neuropsychiatric complications in burn patients. Int J Psychiatry Med 5:2, 1974

6. Avni J: The severe burns. Adv Psychosom Medicine 10: 57–77, 1980

7. Hughes JR, Cayaffa JJ: Seizures following burns of the skin Review of the literature. Diseases Nervous Systems 34:203, 1973

8. Andreasen NJC, Noyes R, Hartford CE, Browland G, Proctor S: Management of emotional reactions in seriously burned adults. New Engl J Med 286(2): 65–69, 1972

9. Hamburg DA, Adams JE: A perspective on coping behavior. Arch Gen Psychiatry 17:277–284, 1967

10. Cobb S, Lindermann E: Neuropsychiatric observations. J Surg 117(6):814–824, 1943

11. Hamburg DC et al: Clinical importance of emotional problems in the care of patients with burns. New Engl J Med 248:355, 1953

12. Klein RM, Charlton JE: Behavioral observation and analysis of pain behavior in critically burned patients. Pain 9:27–40, 1980

13. Quinley S, Bernstein NR: Identity problems and the adaptation of nurses to severely burned children. Am J. Psychiatry 128(1):58–63, 1971

14. Noyes R, Andreasen NJC, Hartford CE: The psychological reaction to severe burns. Psychosomatics 12: 416–422, 1971

15. Kubler-Ross E: On Death & Dying. New York Macmillan, 1969

16. West DA, Shuck JM: Emotional problems of the severely burned patient. Surg Clin North Am 58(6):1189–1204, 1978

17. Imbus SH, Zawacki BE: Autonomy for burned patients when survival is unprecedented. New Engl J Med 297:308–311, 1977

18. Analgesia for Burnt Patients: A Symposium. Br Med J 418–419, 20 May 1972

19. Thal ER, Montgomery SJ, Atkins JM, Roberts BG: Self-administered analgesia with nitrous oxide. JAMA 242(22):2418–2419, 1979

20. Wakeman RJ, Kaplan JZ: An experimental study of hypnosis in painful burns. Am J Clin Hypn 21(1):3–12, 1978

21. Bird EI, Colborne, GR: Rehabilitation of an electrical burn patient through thermal biofeedback. Biofeedback Self Regul 5(2):283–287, 1980

22. Varni JW, Bessman CA, Russo DC, Cataldo MF: Behavioral management of chronic pain in children: case study. Arch Phys Med Rehabil 61:375–379, 1980

23. Mattsson EI: Psychological aspects of severe physical injury and its treatment. J Trauma 15(3):217–234, 1975

24. Steiner H, Clark WR: Psychiatric complications of burned adults: a classification. J Trauma 17(2):134–143, 1977

25. Jorgensen JA, Brophy JJ: Psychiatric treatment of severely burned adults. Psychosom 14:331–335, 1973

26. Mlott SR, Lira FT, Miller WC: Psychological assessment of the burn patient. J Clin Psychol 33(2):425–430, 1977

27. Bernstein NR: Medical tragedies in facial burn disfigurement. Psychiatric Annals 6(10):475–483, 1976

28. MacGregor FC, et al.: Facial Deformities and Plastic Surgery: A Psychosocial Study. Springfield, Illinois, Charles C. Thomas, 1953

29. Solomon JR: Care and needs in a children's burn unit. Prog Pediatr Surg 14:19–32, 1981

30. Molinaro JR: The social fate of children disfigured by burns. Am J Psychiatry 135(8):979–980, 1978

31. McHugh ML, Dimitroff K, Davis ND: Family support group in a burn unit. Am J Nurs 79(12):2148–2150, 1979

6 | Treatment of Burns of Specific Areas

Jean LeMaster

In this chapter we will concentrate on the treatment of burns of specific areas and the particular problems that therapists may encounter. Much of this information may have been covered in other chapters; emphasis in this chapter will be on the significance of injuries to specialized structures. Of course, burns or complications are rarely isolated to a specific area or system, but must be viewed in terms of the totality of the patient.

CARDIOPULMONARY INVOLVEMENT

Cardiopulmonary complications in the burn patient can cause life-threatening situations any time during the course of burn treatment. The likelihood of these complications occurring can be anticipated by taking into consideration the direct injury to the cardiopulmonary system, the extent of the burn injury as a whole, and the past medical history of the patient. Emphasis should be placed on preventive treatment, which can be provided through evaluation of the patient's present cardiopulmonary complications and consideration of the likelihood of possible complications during the course of treatment.

Pulmonary Complications

Pulmonary complications may be divided into those that occur immediately or within the first 48 hours after the burn and those that are delayed. *Immediate* insults to the pulmonary system can be the result of injury from inhalation of smoke, chemicals or steam, high voltage electrical injury, or respiratory response to the burn injury. *Delayed* pulmonary complications include late response to inhalation injury and subsequent pulmonary insufficiency due to the multiple factors of treatment, such as immobilization, pain, sepsis, malnutrition, metabolism, fluid and electrolyte imbalance, aspiration, and the administration of inhalation anesthetics or narcotics.

Pathophysiology and Early Treatment. Immediate life-threatening pulmonary insufficiency can occur at the scene of the burn. In fact, the majority of burn victims who die immediately after injury suffer acute pulmonary deaths. At the injury site, the patient may require cardiopulmonary resuscitation because of respiratory arrests from high voltage electrical injury or from severe hypoxemia due to inhalation of chemicals or the combustion products of smoke. Patients with severe inhalation injury exhibit respiratory distress upon hospital admission.

Physical examination of the patient and the history of the circumstances of the burn injury are clues to the diagnosis of pulmonary pathology. Respiratory complications are probable if the patient exhibits soot in the nose or mouth, singed nasal vibrissae, carbonaceous sputum, hoarseness, stridor, dyspnea, erythema of the mucosa of the nose and mouth, facial burns around the nose and mouth, or tight circumferential burn eschar of the neck and chest. During the emergent phase, edema of the neck can interfere with function of the trachea by compression; and constricting eschar of the neck and chest may inhibit normal excursion of the trachea and thorax. In the patient with severe burn injury (more than 40 percent total body surface area), abdominal distention from paralytic ileus can also compromise disphragmatic excursions, leading to respiratory insufficiency.[1]

Endotracheal intubation may be required when there is tracheal obstruction caused either by edema of the airway structures from a severe inhalation injury or due to edema of the neck. Continuous positive airway pressure with humidified oxygen or mechanical ventilation may be instituted. Tracheostomy is rarely needed during the acute stage unless endotracheal intubation is unsuccessful or associated injuries, such as facial fractures, leave no alternative to this procedure.

Plumonary edema and pneumonia are serious pulmonary complications that can occur as early as eight hours after the burn injury, or after many weeks. Pulmonary edema may result from initial alveoli damage, increased capillary permeability, excessive fluid replacement, or congestive heart failure. Pneumonia may be due to the decreased ability of the damaged respiratory tract cilia to clear bacteria or pulmonary secretions with subsequent occlusion of bronchioles from tracheobronchial debris, causing airway closure, collapse of the alveoli, and bacterial invasion of pooled secretions.

Atelectasis, or collapse of lung segments, can occur any time during the course of burn treatment. Factors contributing to hypoventilation and subsequent atelectasis are airway damage from inhalation injury, poor positioning leading to pooling of secretions, immobilization, and obtunding medication. If secretions cannot be cleared, bacterial growth in these secretions may result in pneumonia.

Physical Therapy Evaluation and Treatment of the Pulmonary Injury. The physical therapy chest evaluation of the burn patient should be comprehensive. A past medical history that includes smoking, prior pulmonary compromise, hypertension, or heart disease may indicate an unfavorable prognosis when combined with inhalation injury and a severe burn. The preinjury nutritional status and the level of physical activity can be indicators of the general strength and cardiopulmonary condition of the patient. Obesity can contribute to decreased diaphragmatic excursion and can indicate general poor nutrition. Age can be a factor: a very young or elderly patient may need more assistance to prevent pulmonary complications.

During the initial physical examination by the therapist, the patient should be observed for color, anatomical structure of the chest, breathing pattern, cough intensity, sputum production, and the presence of adventitious breath sounds. The present mental status should be noted. Associated injuries, such as fractures, which decrease mobility, can adversely affect pulmonary function.

The preinjury respiratory status can affect the treatment. The patient with a recent history of upper respiratory infection or pneumonia should receive continued treatment for these illnesses and should be observed closely for signs of decreasing pulmonary function. Patients with chronic obstructive pulmonary disease (COPD) should be treated for this condition simultaneously with burn and inhalation injury treatment. Medications, such as bronchodilators and expectorants, may be needed to continue to decrease bronchospasm and aid in the clearing of secretions.

Burns of the face, neck, chest, and upper extremities do have an influence on the pulmonary status by hindering movement, chest expansion, and the clearing of pulmonary secretions. Painful nares and lips can reduce the patient's motivation to clear secretions, which in turn can obstruct nasal and oral passages, thus reducing air flow. When the upper extremities are injured and the patient cannot use his hands, all of the secretions produced may not be expectorated.

Decreased chest expansion leading to hypoventilation of the alveoli and atelectasis is a major concern in preventive treatment and has many causes. Complications such as sepsis, metabolic and electrolyte imbalance, hypermetabolism, and malnutrition may result in changes in capillary permeability, shallow breathing, and general muscular weakness. Functional immobility due to pain, depression, medications, and anesthetic administration can result in minimal physical activity and poor lung field expansion. Aspirations of fluids or solid foods in the debilitated patient can occlude airways, leading to alveolar collapse and pneumonia.

Physical therapy treatment of pulmonary complications should begin as soon as possible. The head of the bed should be elevated to ease the work of breathing and decrease edema. If the patient has been placed on mechanical ventilation, he should be assisted in ventilating the lung fields and clearing secretions through the use of postural drainage percussion, vibration, and endotracheal suctioning. When the patient has been extubated or mechanical ventilation removed, the use of incentive spirometry devices, deep breathing exercises, coughing, and increased activity can help maintain adequate ventilation.

Daily decisions regarding treatment should be made in accordance with patient evaluation. Vital signs and chest roentgenograms should be reviewed. Auscultation of the chest for adventitious breath sounds should be performed routinely to direct treatment toward the affected pulmonary segments. If postural drainage is indicated and the involved segment is beneath the burn wound, percussion and vibration over the area will be painful. Therefore, percussion and vibration treatments should be coordinated with the administration of pain medication and the patient given repeated reassurance, as this treatment is uncomfortable and may at times be frightening to the patient.

During these treatments, changes in the patient's mentation, color, breathing

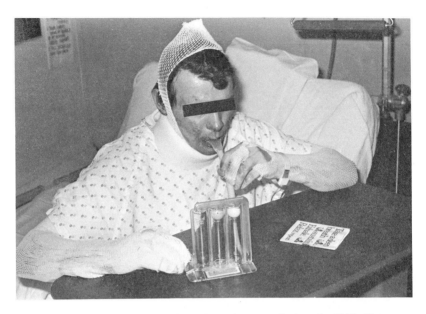

Fig. 6-1.   Patient using incentive spirometry device, the Triflo II.

pattern, sputum production, and breath sounds should be noted. Clinical signs such as dyspnea, increased sputum production, and adventitious breath sounds may indicate a deterioration of the pulmonary status when correlated with increased temperature and a rise in pulse rate. At this time more rigorous physical therapy treatment should be instituted to avert further deterioration. The elderly, uncooperative, or debilitated patient should be observed closely for failing pulmonary function throughout hospitalization.

The physical therapist can teach and supervise deep breathing exercises (to ease the work of breathing), coughing techniques, and adequate clearing of secretions. An incentive spirometry device used hourly by the patient will aid in the performance of sustained maximal inspiration (Fig. 6-1). At all times, the treatment should be coordinated with the nursing and medical staff, as comprehensive pulmonary care is the responsibility of all burn team members and must be carried out 24 hours a day. Education of the patient and patient's family about possible pulmonary complications and the need for frequent lung expansion can help increase motivation and cooperation.

After severe inhalation injury, complications can continue to occur after hospitalization. If there is damage to the vocal cords, hoarseness and vocal cord nodes have to be treated. Whitener et al. have documented decreased vital capacity in pulmonary function tests taken during and after inhalation injury treatment.[4] When a tracheostomy has been performed, tracheal stenosis can be a life-threatening complication. The patient who has had an inhalation injury with a surface burn can be evaluated in the outpatient clinic for respiratory problems as well as for body burn sequelae.

Cardiac Complications

Burn patients may have preinjury cardiac conditions or suffer cardiac complications as a result of the burn injury. Preinjury cardiac conditions that can influence the course of the burn illness include congenital and acquired heart disease, most commonly arteriosclerotic heart disease leading to congestive failure, myocardial infarction, or arrhythmias. Myocardial damage rarely occurs directly from the burn injury, but more commonly, indirectly as a function of anoxia and low flow states. A severe burn injury can lead to arrhythmias as a result of metabolic changes, congestive heart failure, or endocarditis.

The middle-aged or elderly patients with risk factors associated with coronary artery disease may be considered to be at high risk for cardiac complications during treatment. Some contributing factors are obesity, preinjury sedentary activities, smoking, hypertension, and a family history of heart disease. The patient with severe burn injury and real or suspected cardiac involvement generally has a poorer prognosis than others and requires more diligent evaluation and treatment.

As in all situations, physical therapy treatment must be adjusted to the patient's general condition. Adaptation of the patient to exercise is dependent upon age, sex, nutrition, prior physical condition, burn injury complications, and psychological status. Some cardiovascular indicators of exercise tolerance that may be useful in establishing an exercise program are resting pulse rate, respiratory rate and rhythm, blood pressure, electrocardiogram readings, color, disphoresis, and dyspnea. These considerations, combined with the patient's subjective comments, can determine whether the level of exercise that has been initiated should be continued at the present level or in some way altered.

A progressive cardiovascular conditioning program should be incorporated into the rehabilitation of all burn patients. Patients with documented cardiac conditions and poor exercise response should be monitored during the exercise program, and this program progressed according to the patient's condition and response. Cardiovascular fitness can continue to be improved by a posthospitalization activity program coupled with weight and smoking reduction suggestions.

BURNS OF THE FACE AND SCALP

Burns of the face and scalp are difficult and frustrating management problems for all members of the burn team. Even with excellent wound care, contracture, which occurs with wound healing and grafting in deep facial burns, may result in severe disfigurement and functional loss. Pressure therapy can decrease contracture and hypertrophic scarring, but cannot alleviate change in appearance that the burn patient suffers. Emotional support given with meticulous wound care can help decrease the psychological and physical sequelae of deep facial and scalp burns.

Special Areas of Concern: Eyes, Nose, Mouth, and Ears

Edema occurring during the emergent phase following severe burn injury to the head may interfere with respiratory function, vision, nutrition, and may possibly contribute to cerebral edema and seizure activity in children. The head of the bed should be elevated to help decrease edema. Acute management of the burn injury to these areas includes daily observation of the wound, shaving of all hair around the injury (except for the eyebrows), daily cleansing of the wounds and surrounding area, careful debridement of eschar and exudate, and the application of topical agents and dressings. Areas of the head that require special attention are eyes, nose, mouth, and ears. Each area has distinct wound care needs as well as skin contracture conse-quences, which occur quickly with wound healing.

During the emergent phase, antibiotic ointments should be applied to edematous eyes to prevent infection.[5] If there is corneal damage, the use of eye patches, medi-cation to the cornea, or irrigation may be warranted. Ectropion or eversion of the eyelids, can and frequently does occur from skin contracture of burns of the eyelids. Such contracture may prevent adequate covering of the cornea and result in corneal desiccation and, ultimately, infection and blindness. The application of artificial tears may be needed to prevent corneal drying until definitive eyelid reconstruction pro-cedures provides coverage. If this is unsatisfactory, tarsorrhaphy, or suturing of the eyelids, may be necessary. After an electrical injury, cataracts are possible, although rarely a complication.

The nose, with its complex three-dimensional characteristics and only a thin cover of soft tissue, is very susceptible to infection and ultimate loss of definitive contour. Daily cleansing and general debridement will reduce the possibility of infec-tion and cartilage loss. Debris should be cleaned from the nares to facilitate normal respiratory function. With healing, skin contracture can result in the downward, or lateral, pull of the nostrils, thereby producing cosmetic deformities and obstructing airflow through the nares. An orthotic device may be inserted into the nares to main-tain the shape of the ala and allow adequate air flow.

Good oral hygiene is required of both the burned and unburned mouth to mini-mize the possibility of superinfection. The patient should be instructed and assisted in proper mouth care. If the lips are burned, topical cream or ointment can be applied to encourage epithelialization, prevent desiccation, and prevent the development of unfavorable crusts. In oral and perioral burns, microstomia, or contracture of the mouth, can begin early in the healing process and, if allowed to progress, may inter-fere with oral hygiene, nutrition, the administration of anesthesia, and cause undesir-able aesthetic consequences. Contractures around the lips and nasolabial area can cause eversion of the lips with inability to close the mouth.

The ear is particularly susceptible to damage from thermal injury because of its exposed position and its very thin, soft tissue covering. The ear is a complex mass of convolutions and contours, and once destroyed, can rarely be restored to an ac-ceptable appearance. Meticulous wound care is needed to cleanse the uneven sur-faces. If dressings are applied to the ear, gauze should be placed in the complex contours to help maintain the shape of the ear, and also placed between the temporal bone and the auricle to prevent maceration and contracture of that particularly vul-nerable skin. Exposed cartilage should have wet antimicrobial dressings applied to it until it is well-healed. Chondritis, or infection of the cartilage, is a common compli-cation produced from fracture and exposure of the auricular cartilage. This compli-cation demands immediate surgical intervention and debridement. Until there is complete coverage of the ear, the patient, to avoid lying on and fracturing the delicate auricular cartilage, should not be allowed to use a pillow.

Late Consequences of Facial Burns

Distorting contractures of the eyelids, nose, mouth, and ears coupled with contracture of adjacent facial skin can lead to severe disfigurement and functional loss (Fig. 6-2). Disfigurement results from the contracting scar distorting normal facial features. When hypertrophic scarring occurs, the extent of this distortion is amplified. Functional complications can include inability to close the eyes, loss of facial expression, teeth malalignment, drooling and inability to close the lips, and difficulty in speaking, breathing, and eating. Facial exercises and the application of orthotic and pressure devices can help minimize, but not prevent, facial complications.

Facial exercises should be started immediately after injury and be continued until wound maturation, which may be six to twelve months posthospital discharge. Facial exercises should include the full range of all facial muscle groups. Coordinating facial and neck exercises can provide long scar stretches of the combined facial and neck area, thus extending the effects of the stretch.

Orthotic devices and pressure therapy using elastic and/or rigid materials can aid in the prevention and reduction of contracture in hypertrophic scarring of the facial skin. In perioral burns, an orthotic device may be needed to prevent or correct microstomia. This device can be applied soon after burn injury and should be worn until wound maturation. The extent of the daily use of the device is determined by

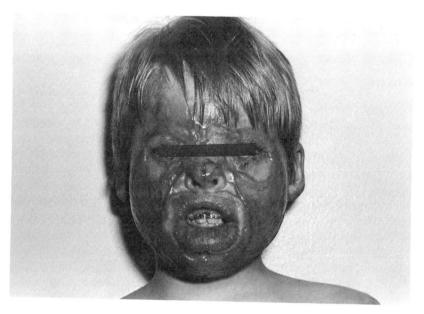

Fig. 6-2. Contracture and hypertrophic scarring of the face, causing severe facial distortion. Note dense hypertrophic scarring, ectropian of the lower lids, and eversion of the lips.

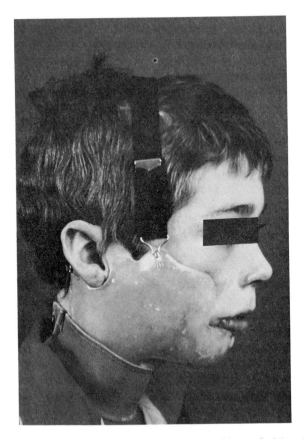

Fig. 6-3. A partial plastic transparent face mask to control lower facial and neck scarring.

the degree of contracture: patients with severe microstomia must wear it continuously, whereas those with minimal contracture may require it only at night.

Depending upon the location of the burn, commercially made or custom-fitted elastic face masks or chin straps can be ordered. Because the elastic mask tends to bridge the nose and perioral regions, inserts of silicon or thermoplastic material can be used in these difficult areas. The elastic face mask also conceals the facial features and scalp, and many patients find it cosmetically unacceptable, which results in problems with patient compliance. A custom-made transparent plastic facial mask can provide adequate pressure and eliminate some of the unacceptable features of elastic masks Fig. 6-3.[6] To properly fabricate and fit this mask requires training and practice. When made from moulages of the patient's face, good scar contact with the mask is possible. If needed, this rigid mask can be altered to accommodate an orthotic device used to prevent microstomia. Pressure therapy to the face can be commenced 10 to 14 days after facial scar healing, and the mask should be worn continuously until skin maturation.

With most facial burns that require hospitalization, there are changes in the facial skin texture, color, and lubrication, which continues at least until the injured area has matured, or perhaps indefinitely. Patients with healed facial burns often complain of skin eruptions, dryness or oiliness of the skin, hypersensitivity to sunlight or cold, and folliculitis or inflammation of hair follicles of the beard in men. In order to minimize these complications, frequent cleansing and a thorough rinsing of the facial skin is recommended along with the judicious application of lubricating lotions. The application of sun screen lotions and the use of broad brimmed hats during periods of sun, exposure, and the wearing of ski masks during time of cold exposure is sometimes helpful in protecting scar tissue. If orthotic pressure devices or elastic garments are being used for scar control, they should be cleansed and dried before application. If facial reconstructive procedures are needed for cosmetic or functional reasons, reapplication of these pressure devices or garments after such operations may be needed. Custom prosthetic devices are sometimes utilized to replace partial or complete loss of facial features such as nose or ears.

Burns of the Scalp

Thermal injury of the scalp and the use of the scalp for donor sites can cause considerable damage. Wound care of partial- and full-thickness scalp burns is complicated by the great density of hair follicles, which may become infected, or by the growth of hair into the exudate and eschar, which makes debridement difficult. Daily shaving of the scalp hair in and around the involved areas can minimize these difficulties. Electrical burn injury and deep contact injury may cause not only full-thick-

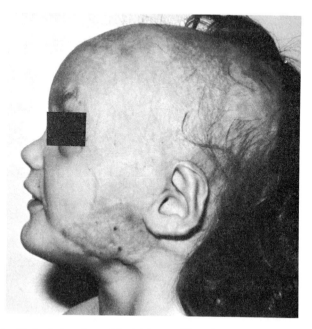

Fig. 6-4. Child with healed scalp and facial burns. Note the less hypertrophic scarring over the convex area of the scalp as compared to the areas of the face.

ness loss of the scalp, but also loss of the underlying bony cranium. Exposed necrotic bone should be surgically removed and burr holes drilled through the remaining cortex to stimulate the production of granulation tissue. Wet dressings should then be applied to the exposed cranium until granulation tissue is sufficient to support autografts. In electrical burns with cranial damage, neurological complications may occur.[7] Initial symptoms are often confusion and irritability, or perhaps seizures with the possible late development of hemiparesis and ataxia. In addition, the patient may complain of chronic headaches.

Folliculitis and chronic ulceration can be a long-term complication of healed scalp burns. However, hypertrophic scarring and contracture of the skin overlying the cranium are surprisingly minimal due to the pressure produced by the pull of the skin over the convex cranium (Fig. 6-4). Baldness following the application of autografts or closure of a cranial defect can be corrected by autogenous hair transplantation. In those patients with bony cranial defects, however, a helmet may be worn for protection until the defect can be corrected. A definitive hairpiece with an acrylic insert can be placed over the cranial defect for improved cosmetic appearance and cranial protection if surgical correction is not possible or delayed.

BURNS OF THE NECK

Acute Phase Considerations

In the emergent phase, the immediate concerns in the care of neck burns are maintenance of a patent airway and the possibility of cervical spine injury. Partial- or full-thickness thermal destruction of the thin, elastic skin of the anterior and lateral surfaces of the neck can occur quickly. Subsequent edema formation beneath a partial-thickness neck burn or the constricting eschar of a full-thickness circumferential neck burn can compress the underlying trachea, causing upper airway obstruction. Endotracheal intubation and/or escharotomy of constricting full-thickness neck eschar may be needed to relieve this obstruction. The head of the bed should be elevated to decrease breathing effort and to minimize edema formation. Circumferential dressings or the use of neck orthases should not be initiated until edema subsides and adequate respiratory function has been established.

If the burn injury is produced by electrical contact, explosion, or motor vehicle accident, then cervical fracture and/or spinal cord injury is a possibility. Evaluation of neurological signs and roentgenographic examination can determine the presence and extent of the injury to the cervical vertebrae. A fracture of the cervical spine, with or without spinal cord injury, may require immobilization and/or immediate surgical intervention to establish spinal stability.

Evaluation and Treatment

Evaluation of the patient with neck burns should include the circumstances of the burn, evaluation of the cervical spine, past medical history, age, mental status, and the depth and location of the burns of the neck and adjacent areas. The circum-

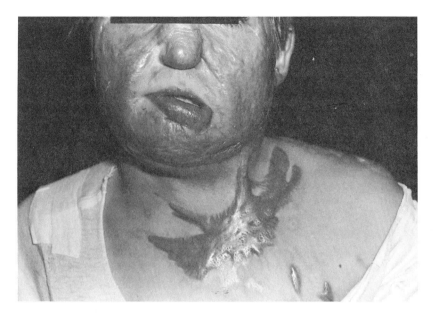

Fig. 6-5. Unilateral neck burn causing disfigurement of the lower facial features and limited cervical range of motion.

stances of the burn injury can indicate the possible occurrence of an inhalation injury or cervical spine injury. Past medical history, that may include arthritis, degenerative disc disease, or surgical procedures, can influence surgical range of motion and patient comfort. The age and mental status of the patient will aid in predicting compliance with the treatment program. The very young, confused, or elderly patient may need assistance in completing the treatment regimen.

Location and depth of the burns of the neck and adjacent areas can influence wound healing sequence. A full-thickness burn injury will necessitate immobilization for autografting procedures. Deep partial- or full-thickness burns are more likely to develop contractures and hypertrophic scarring than superficial injuries. Anterior and lateral neck contractures joined with skin contractures of the face and chest can cause lower lip eversion, loss of normal cervical spine range of motion, limited visual fields, malalignment of teeth, and difficulty in the administration of anesthesia (Fig. 6-5). Posterior neck contractures can increase cervical lordosis, thereby interfering with the patient's normal postural pattern. Neck, chest, and upper extremity skin contractures often combine to limit horizontal abduction of the upper extremities and can produce postural changes, such as scapular protraction, elevation of the shoulders, and kyphosis.

Treatment of neck burns should include good wound care, proper positioning, neck exercises, and use of neck orthotics and pressure garments. Daily cleansing, debridement, and application of topical agents and dressings to the affected areas can help prevent infection and promote early wound healing. Proper positioning of the neck should be initiated immediately after hospital admission. Pillows should not be used because they encourage flexion of the neck, obstruction of the airway, and contracture of the anterior and lateral neck burns. Therefore, a small foam pad, which allows minimal flexion of the cervial spine, should be placed beneath the head instead of a pillow. This foam pad can also aid in patient comfort and the prevention of decubiti of the scalp. The use of a foam pad should be continued until there is no longer a risk of neck contracture. Proper alignment in positioning of the head, neck, and trunk of the patient can help prevent poor postural habits.

The patient should perform full range and active flexion, extension, and rotation of the cervical spine during the acute phase of burn injury. This program should continue until scar maturation is complete. To allow for graft adherence following autograft procedures, exercise should be discontinued for three to five days following the surgical procedure. To avoid injury to the cervical spine, care should be taken when assisting in neck exercises in patients with a past history of decreased cervical spine mobility, patients over 40 years of age, or patients in pain.

Combining neck extension and rotation exercises with facial exercises can stretch advancing anterior and lateral neck skin contractures and increase cervical range of motion. Forward flexion exercises of the neck can stretch posterior neck contractures, thus helping to prevent increased cervical lordosis. Neck and trunk extension mat exercises combined with upper extremity exercises can improve mobility of the neck, thorax, and upper extremity scars.

The application of neck orthosis and pressure garments can aid in the prevention of neck contractures. The neck orthoses should be applied while the wound is healing, and continued until complete scar maturation. Immobilization after autografting procedures may be accomplished by positioning either with or without neck orthesis.[8,9] Mandibular skeletal traction has been used for immobilization of neck autografts, but is not recommended in children because of the possibility of damage to the epiphyseal cartilage of the mandible.[10] It usually takes seven to ten days after autograft application to assure sufficient graft integrity to allow the use of a definitive neck orthosis or pressure garment.

The rigid neck orthosis used during the acute and rehabilitative phases of burn injury treatment was introduced by Willis.[11] This splint is made of thermoplastic material and is fabricated directly on the patient. The process of splint fabrication may be difficult and painful. Special training in the fabrication and fitting of the splints is necessary. Since its inception, the thermoplastic neck splint has been modified to eliminate the high mandibular section that previously caused mandibular and teeth malalignment.

Another type of rigid splint is the custom-made acrylic or plastic orthosis. This splint is made by following the same fabrication principles as in the transparent face mask—the use of a moulage.

The single piece foam neck orthosis can be utilized during the acute and rehabilitative phase for the prevention of scar contractures. This foam collar does not require any particular expertise in fabrication, and is more comfortable than the rigid splint. Some centers have found the use of multiple foam rings helpful. One or more circumferential neck rings can be added or removed as neck contracture increases or decreases.

Pressure to neck scar is generally applied through an orthosis. In addition, the

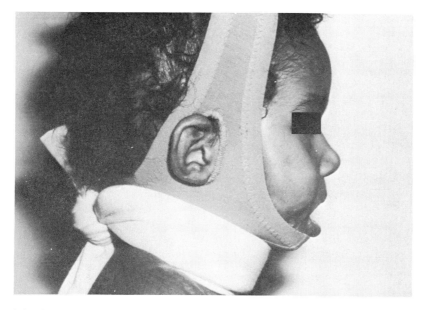

Fig. 6-6.   Use of elastic chin strap to control hypertrophic scarring of lower face and foam neck collar to minimize neck flexion contracture.

extension of pressure to adjacent burned areas is needed for effective scar control. A combination of transparent or elastic face masks with a neck orthosis may be used when facial burn injury has occurred in association with thermal injury to the neck. Elastic chin straps applied in conjunction with neck collars may help decrease scarring of the lateral and lower face areas, jawline, and neck (Fig. 6-6). Pressure vests with turtle neck extensions may help to control upper chest scarrings when used with a neck orthosis.

In established neck contractures, reconstructive surgical procedures are required for correction of inadequate neck contour and limited range of motion. Neck orthoses, which will be needed after these surgical procedures to maintain the chin/neck angle, should be fabricated preoperatively. Use of neck orthoses is especially indicated when split-thickness skin grafts are to be applied. Splinting over the area of contracture release and subsequent grafting is usually necessary for three to six months after release.

BURNS OF THE HAND AND WRIST

Significant burns of the hand affect physical, social, psychological, and economic aspects of the patient's life. Although the skin of the hand comprises a relatively minor portion of the total body surface, its sensitivity allows complex movements of the fingers, which permit grasp and manipulation of objects and a tactile link with our environment. Biomechanical impairment and loss of the normal cosmetic appearance of the hand can influence the patient's self-image as well as his occupation and of lifestyle.

Pathophysiology

Functional loss of the burned hand and wrist can result from damage or loss of anatomical structures, persistent edema, faulty positioning, and contracture and hypertrophy of the resulting scar. The thin, elastic skin of the dorsum of the hand is more likely to suffer a full-thickness burn injury than the thick, inflexible skin of the palmar surface. During the accident, burn victims usually flex their fingers, thus protecting the thick palmar skin and exposing the thinner dorsal skin to damage. Skin elasticity, independence of the tissue layers, and lymphatic composition allow for the accumulation of edema in the dorsum of the hand. Because critically important anatomical structures lie close to the skin of the dorsal aspect of the hand, the potential for functional loss as a result of this edema is great. Damage to anatomical structures in the palm usually occur only as a result of a charring injury, direct contact, or electrical burn.

Electrical and severe burn injury may immediately damage hand anatomy or have serious delayed consequences. During the emergent period, both injuries can cause severe edema or constricting eschar, which can lead to vascular compression and further progressive ischemia. The injuries may also directly damage the vascular supply in the proximal aspect of the upper extremity. Electrical injuries may lead to full-thickness skin loss of the hand or complete destruction of viable tissue, requiring amputation.[12] The clinical consequences of electrical damage to the muscular, vascular, and neural systems are often manifested late in electrical injuries.

Skin contracture and hypertrophic scarring can occur on both the dorsal and palmar surfaces of the hand, although it is much more common in the more vulnerable dorsal surface. The normal elastic, versatile skin of the dorsum can be replaced by burn scar, which is immobile and constrictive. The tight scar can contribute to hyperextension deformity of the metacarpophalangeal (MP) joint, especially of the ring and little fingers. Contracture of the thumb and finger web spaces can decrease precision prehension and cylindrical grasp. A contracted scar overlying the thenar and hypothenar eminences uniting with a scar of the volar surface of the wrist can limit finger and wrist extension. When tendon and bone are exposed, there may be adherence of the scar to these structures, resulting in limitation of movement.

Deformities of the hand can involve single or multiple joints and often develop because of musculotendinous imbalance and scar or joint contracture. The most common deformities that result when contracture prevention procedures have failed, are hyperextension of the MP joints, flexion of the interphalangeal (IP) joints, flattening of the transverse and longitudinal palmar arches, adduction of the thumb, and volar flexion of the wrist (Fig. 6-7).

In the dorsal burn injury of the thin skin overlying the proximal interphalangeal (PIP) joint, rupture of the extensor hood and interruption of the central slip of the extensor digitorum communis tendon commonly leads to the boutonniere deformity of the finger. This deformity consists of MP hyperextension, PIP joint flexion, and DIP joint hyperextension with loss of function of the central slip of the extensor

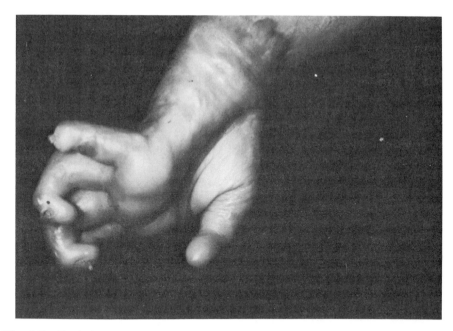

Fig. 6-7.   Typical contracture deformity of a hand burn in a child. Note the hyperextension deformity of the MCP joints, especially those of the little and ring finger.

tendon, volar displacement of the lateral bands of the extensor tendon, and secondary contracture of the joint capsule and volar plate. If MP joint hyperextension is not corrected, the collateral ligaments can shorten, thus restricting MP joint mobility. Postthermal injury boutonniere deformity of the PIP joint is, unfortunately, quite common and very difficult to correct.

Prolonged finger joint deformity will ultimately cause imbalance of the long flexor and extensor muscles and tightness of the intrinsic muscles. Due to the lax collateral ligamentous structure of the thumb carpometacarpal joint, contracture of the palm may result in dislocation at the first carpometacarpal joint. Other deformities that may develop in hand and wrist burns are swan-neck deformities, flexion deformities of the fingers, interdigital syndactyly, little finger abduction and rotation, hyperextension of the thumb IP joint, and radial wrist deviation (Fig. 6-8).

Acute Phase Considerations

Evaluation and appropriate treatment of thermal injuries of the hand depends upon the depth and location of the injury, knowledge of potential wound healing sequelae, and treatment methods. These factors are modified in each case by the individual patient characteristics and compliance. The immediate concerns in the emergent phase are edema formation and possible vascular impairment. If there is vascular impairment from edema or constricting eschar, midlateral escharotomies may

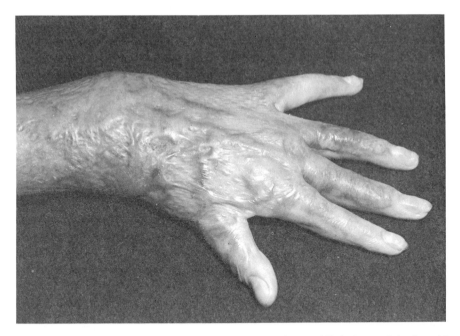

Fig. 6-8.   Hand deformities of wrist flexion, radial deviation, and little finger abduction. Also note a contracture of thumb web space and volar drift of the web spaces of the digits.

be needed. Doppler examination may determine the presence of inadequate blood flow to the distal portions of the finger.

Edema, wound healing, joint integrity, and muscular and neural functions should be assessed daily. Since the skin of the hand dorsum is thin, care should be taken during debridement to prevent damage to the underlying extensor hood over the PIP joint. Removal of eschar and exudate crusts around fingernails can help prevent fingerpulp infection, which can delay finger use in activities in daily living. Exposed tendon and bone should have wet dressings continuously applied to avoid desiccation and further damage to these structures. Individual finger and palmar dressings rather than bulky, mitten-type dressings can facilitate hand movement during this difficult phase.

Skeletal fixation is a controversial method used for positioning and immobilization of burns of the hands and wrist. In these burns, skeletal fixation involves placement of transverse or intramedullary Kirschner wires through the phalanges and a Steinmann pin in the radius. The hand is then suspended from an apparatus over the patient's bed. Achauer et al. advocated the use of skeletal fixation in patients with hand burns in order to prevent deformity.[13] Alexander et al. found that the use of intramedullary Kirschner wires, following reconstructive procedures for finger deformities, did not increase autograft take or the long-term functional results.[14] Proper care must always be taken at the pin sites to avoid wound infections and possible osteomyelitis. In complicated fractures and dislocations, skeletal fixation may be necessary for bony alignment and for exposure of the burn wound to facilitate wound care.

Skeletal fixation is a temporary immobilization method requiring, after its removal, an additional method of hand positioning to continue contracture prevention. External splinting and the use of skeletal fixation can only prevent joint impairment if properly applied and carefully supervised.

Active exercises of the fingers and wrist can help to maintain muscle awareness, prevent tendon adhesions, and maintain the length of muscular and ligamentous tissue. The patient who is unable to perform full active range of motion should be assisted in attaining this goal. In the acute phase, emphasis should be directed to MP joint flexion, IP extension, thumb extension and abduction, and wrist extension. Exercises of the entire upper extremity should be included within the total hand program. Performance of full range of motion exercises and rigorous attention to the position of the hand and wrist can often prevent edema and joint deformity during the acute phase of the burn injury, thus reducing the need for splinting and allowing for patient freedom of motion.[15,16,17]

If there is involvement of the extensor hood of the PIP joint, immobilization of this joint is recommended until wound healing has occurred in order to prevent further tendon damage. Throughout treatment, the patient can improve mobility by using the hands in activities of daily living (ADLs), such as eating and transferring. Posting a list of exercises in the patient's room and including the patient's family in the supervision of ADLs and the exercise program can be of help. Following autografts, movement should be restricted for three to five days to allow for graft adherence. After this time, active exercises should be progressed rapidly to regain range of motion.

Proper hand and joint positioning should begin as soon as possible in the emergent period in order to avoid dependent edema and to prevent joint deformity. Correct positioning can be accomplished with pillows or foam support, or by immobilization with external splinting devices or skeletal traction. Because of the lymphatic impairment that accompanies deep dorsal hand burns, evaluation of the hand is necessary throughout hospitalization to prevent edema formation. Extreme flexion of the wrist should be avoided to prevent overstretching of the radial nerve and possible subsequent neuropathy. Extreme extension of the wrist can lead to median and ulnar nerve neuropathies.

Several types of splints are available for hand and wrist positioning. Hand and wrist splints made of low temperature thermoplastic materials are frequently applied when the patient is unable to maintain proper hand positioning or after surgical procedures. The volar extension splint can help prevent deformity by providing wrist support, which maintains appropriate flexor and extensor muscular length and frees the fingers and thumb for active use. Individual finger extension splints can decrease trauma to exposed PIP joints, as well as maintain tendinous and ligamentous length until wound healing or definitive surgical correction. Specialized splints may be required to provide immobilization after autografts or support fractures and dislocations. Central or peripheral nerve injuries may require assistive devices to minimize hand dysfunction. During all phases of treatment, caution should be taken in the use of circular bandages or straps, which may produce distal circulatory compromise.

Rehabilitative Phase Considerations

Rehabilitation of the severely burned hand is a long and complex task complicated by scar contracture, scar hypertrophy, activity limitations, sensory changes, and psychological maladaptation. Scar contracture and hypertrophy can cause motions to be less flexible and spontaneous even when range of motion of individual joints appears normal. The unsightly appearance of the hand can affect the patient's body image as well as his/her interpersonal relationships. Functional and cosmetic impairment can be iminmized through a rigorous program of pressure therapy, active exercises, and the use of orthotics.

Pressure Therapy.   Pressure gloves can be applied to the burned hand for scar protection and to decrease hypertrophic scarring. The glove should be ordered when the hand is nearly healed, and applied, if tolerated, as early as ten days after complete epithelialization. If there is residual edema in the hand, measurements should not be taken for custom-made gloves. Cotton elastic gloves of standard sizes can be applied until the size of the hand has stabilized (Fig. 6-9). If contractures of the web spaces are present, foam, elastomer, or thermoplastic splint material may be used in web spaces to control contracture.

Splinting.   After healing, splinting may be needed to counteract the strong pull of wound contracture. Most frequently, splints are applied to prevent flexion and rotation deformities of the fingers (Fig. 6-10), adduction webbing of the thumb, and palmar contracture associated with volar contracture of the wrist. Wearing time of the splints depends upon the speed with which the contracture develops. Patient ed-

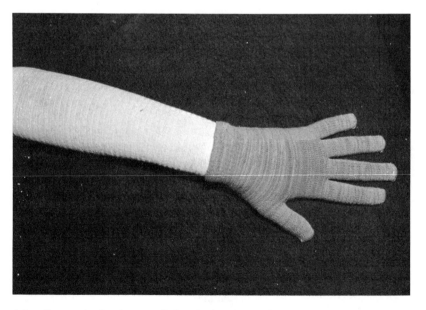

Fig. 6-9.   Cotton elastic glove applied to healed burned hand and tubular pressure bandage applied to the forearm.

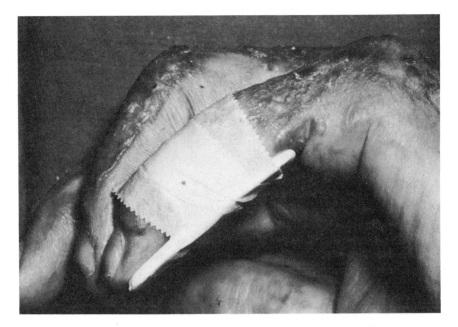

Fig. 6-10.   Extension splint applied to little finger to prevent flexion of PIP joint. Care must be taken in application to avoid injury to delicate, recently epithelialized skin.

ucation regarding scar evaluation and prevention will enable many patients to adjust the splint wearing time according to their changing needs. Dynamic splinting has been successful in the correction of long-term contractures of the finger and in providing a functional aid in peripheral and central nerve injuries. Use of this type of splint is limited, as it requires scar tolerance to friction, proper application of the splint by the patient, and availability of the patient and therapist for splint alteration.

Exercise.   The patient who performs exercises well when in the hospital may have difficulty with progressive scar contracture and hypertrophy and decreased joint mobility after hospitalization. Care of each finger joint can become a major problem as the scar opposes normal joint alignment. Involvement of adjacent elbow and shoulder joints can significantly affect the ability to elevate and position the hand properly. Mobility of the wrist is necessary for proper positioning of the hand. Outpatient treatment may be needed for hands-on therapy or for emotional support. For the patient who is unable to return to work quickly, meaningful activities, such as woodworking, combined with hand and wrist exercises can be effective in maintaining joint range of motion and flexibility as well as improving psychological adaptation.

Small unhealed areas and hypersensitivity further complicate therapy in the postthermally injured hand. Small unhealed areas result from abrasion of the newly formed delicate epithelium. Blister formation occurs in areas of friction. These unhealed areas are painful, and healing may be delayed. Loss of papillary ridges and hypersensitivity of fingertips makes performance of the activities of daily living difficult. Because of the sensitivity of the scar, sensory input to the hand in the environment is primarily unpleasant and may further hinder progress. The psychological impact of an unsightly hand, which is difficult and painful to move, can have serious implications in long-term hand function. Ongoing education of the patient and family regarding wound-healing sequelae and possible future treatment can aid in postburn adaptation. Considering the importance of the hand to a person's life, a thorough evaluation of treatment in all aspects of hand care is imperative in promoting normal function.

There are few studies of long-term functional and sensory changes of burn injuries to the hand. Frank et al. and Fissette et al. have reported burn injuries producing nerve entrapment syndromes at the wrist.[18,19] Frank et al. suggest using only slight wrist extension in hand splints to prevent excessive narrowing of the carpal space and possible neural damage. In the patient with diabetes or alcohol dependence, peripheral neuropathies may become evident. Other complications seen after wound healing are muscular weakness, sensory changes, increased sensitivity to heat and cold, and poor psychological acceptance of the hand. In electrical burns with peripheral nerve injury, partial or complete loss of nerve function may require an orthotic aid.

BURNS OF THE EXTREMITIES

The extent of functional morbidity following burns of the extremities is dependent on the joints directly involved in the burn injury and the treatment given to the joints during the acute and rehabilitative phases. Unless there are musculoskeletal and neuromuscular complications, all affected joints are expected to have normal range of motion after burn treatment and physical therapy. Although attention during treatment is directed primarily toward the burned extremities, the unburned extremities should not be neglected.

To develop a treatment plan, a thorough evaluation of the patient is necessary. Past medical history may reveal problems such as arthritis, fractures, trauma, and surgical procedures causing joint pain or loss of range of motion and function. The body type of the patient is an indication of the general flexibility and prior level of activity. The very muscular or obese person frequently does not have the ease of movement seen in the person of thin or medium build. Whether the person was working, sedentary, engaged in recreational exercises, or had an alcohol or drug dependency prior to injury will help to predict the discipline and motivation of the patient. The young or elderly patient, the patient with a psychiatric disorder, and the patient with low pain tolerance may have a lack of comprehension or ability to comply with therapy. A thorough evaluation of all extremities includes a notation of amounts of edema, present range of motion, associated injuries such as fractures or dislocations, nervous system damage, and location and depth of the burn. Destruction of anatomical structures and possible neurological damage can be anticipated in the patient with electrical, severe flame, or contact injuries.

A well-supervised daily treatment plan adapted to individual patients can prevent many complications. Huang et al. found that with the use of contracture prevention procedures, there was a decreased incidence of contractures and frequency and need for corrective surgical procedures in the axilla, elbow, wrist, and knee joints.[20] These procedures, which will prevent contractures and maintain joint range of motion, are positioning, splinting, exercise, and pressure dressings.

Acute Phase Considerations

Treatment of the extremities during the emergent phase is directed toward the prevention of dependent edema and circulatory compromise. Circulatory impairment of distal extremities due to severe edema or constricting eschar may at times be determined by ultrasonic Doppler flowmeter examination. Escharotomy should be performed when the circumferential extremity burn restricts circulation. In electrical burns, fasciotomies are sometimes necessary to restore circulation.

Elevation and early mobilization of the extremity can aid in the prevention of dependent edema. The upper extremities should be elevated to prevent deposition of edema in the elbow area. In the lower extremity, elevation and movement of the foot and ankle will aid mobilization of edema fluid. Extreme elevation of the lower extremities should be avoided because it will only shift obligatory edema to the pelvis and lower abdomen.

Upper Extremity

Burns over multiple joints of the upper extremity can increase potential for functional loss because of the larger surface area of the burn wound itself and because of the greater pain associated with rehabilitative efforts. Contracture deformities of the upper extremity can occur in the hand, wrist, elbow, or shoulder. Patient participation and timing of preventive treatment are most important in attaining a good functional result.

Proper positioning should include shoulder abduction and elbow extension. Extreme shoulder extension with abduction is to be avoided because of possible brachial plexus injury. External or neutral rotation of the shoulder is a goal in upper extremity positioning, but cannot always be maintained when the patient relaxes and as a result of gravity, the extremity assumes a more comfortable position of slight internal rotation with pronation of the forearm. Elbow extension and axillary splints can aid in keeping both elbows and shoulders in the proper position. During the acute phase of injury, prolonged pressure over the posterior elbow may produce pressure ulceration over the olecranon and compression of the ulnar nerve, which may lead to later perpheral neuropathy.

Full shoulder or elbow ROM can be difficult to maintain. Gravity, the greater strength of the flexor muscles, and the patient's tendency to position in flexion in response to pain contribute to shoulder abduction and flow and elbow flexion. As the burn wound heals, the resulting scar contracture coupled with the stronger flexor muscles can make the adverse position of flexion permanent (Fig. 6-11).

Successful rehabilitation of the upper extremity requires the patient's full understanding of the possible functional consequences and his complete participation in treatment programs. Treatments should emphasize *activity* and limit the use of im-

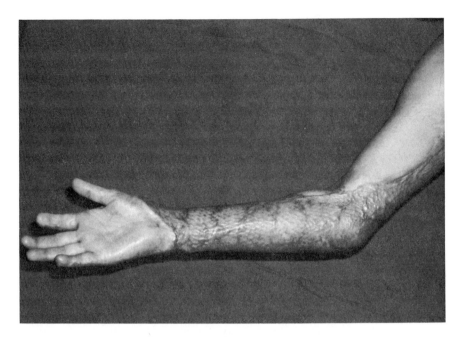

Fig. 6-11.   Upper extremity scarring pattern, which causes elbow flexion contracture. Healed, autografted upper extremity burns, which will tend to produce flexion contracture at elbow and limitation of wrist extension upon elbow extension.

mobilization. After autografting, postoperative immobilization should be minimal (three to five days) before active exercise is reinstated. Exercises using a cane or overhead pulleys can help the patient maintain shoulder motion during the active phase of injury and can be continued during rehabilitation. With healing, the patient can progress to mat exercises, which can include rolling, sit-ups, and push-ups. Dance exercises and meaningful upper extremity activities can improve the patient's flexibility and motivation.

Pressure Garments and Splints.   The use of pressure garments and orthoses in the treatment of upper extremity burns should be guided by an evaluation of the burn wound or healed scar and the patient's tolerance of such devices. Care should be taken when applying pressure or splints in elderly patients, in patients with circulatory compromise, and in patients with severe hand burns, as improperly applied devices can increase morbidity by causing circulatory embarrassment. A figure of eight dressing incorporating foam pads in the axilla and applied with an elastic bandage can be used during and after healing to prevent axillary contractures (Fig. 6-12). This device allows shoulder movement while controlling contracture of the axillary scar. A rigid axilla or axillary orthosis can be applied at night to maintain the length of the axillary folds. In the patient having difficulty with active elbow extension, the use of intermittent splinting will help maintain optimal joint position while avoiding prolonged immobilization. Elastic wrap bandages or cotton tubular bandages are

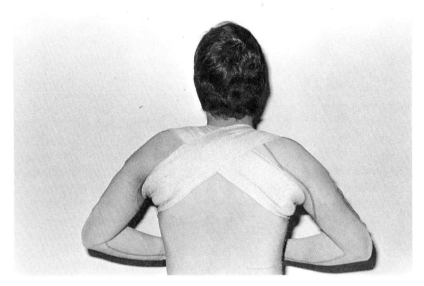

Fig. 6-12. Figure of eight axillary dressing used to prevent axillary contractures. Also note the use of custom-made compression garments.

sometimes used after autografting sessions and before custom-fitted pressure garments become available. Because elastic wraps can be applied with inconsistent pressure, the patient should be evaluated for circulatory compromise after the application. When a few unhealed areas remain, cotton tubular elastic bandage can be applied to begin scar control and protect friable tissue. The number of layers used will depend on the scar and the patient's tolerance. Layers can be increased as circulation and scar adjust to the pressure. If custom-made garments are desired for the upper extremity and trunk, they are ordered when the patient's weight and the size of the extremity has stabilized.

A frequently seen long-term complication of burns of the upper extremity is skin breakdown over the olecranon. It may be necessary to lessen the pressure used to control wound healing over these areas until complete epithelialization has occurred. It may also be helpful to place padding over the olecranon to prevent it from abrasion and further breakdown. If release is needed for either elbow or axillary contractures, postoperative preventive measures, such as extension splints, may be necessary to maintain the length gained from the surgical procedure.

Lower Extremity

Hip contractures, knee inflexion, ankle equines, and toe hyperextension are complications to be avoided in burns of the lower extremity. Hip contractures can be either in adduction and internal rotation or abduction and external rotation, depending on the position the patient assumes when supine. Adverse knee contractures occur in flexion, and adverse toe contractures occur in extension.

Ambulation should commence as soon as possible after hospital admission. Elastic bandages are applied to the lower extremity to aid circulation and decrease the pain that is frequently encountered upon assuming the upright position. When there are burns of the soles of the feet, pads may be placed on the soles to make walking more tolerable. Assistive walking devices are used only if necessary. When the patient is not walking, the lower extremities should be elevated to control edema. Edema may be a recurring probelm in the patient with deep circumferential leg burns or improperly applied elastic bandages, and in the patient with congestive heart failure or fluid and electrolyte imbalance. In some centers, patients with lower extremity burns are not allowed to ambulate until the burn wounds are completely healed.

Many types of pressure devices can be used in the lower extremity with good results. These include elastic wrap bandages, commercially sized elastic stockings, custom-made elastic stockings, and cotton elastic tubular-shaped bandages. The ease of application and comfort to the patient are considerations when determining which type of device is to be applied. Patients with circumferential full-thickness injuries to the legs may wear pressure stockings indefinitely to prevent the occurrence of varicosities and the discomfort that is sometimes experienced when standing. In order to prevent hypertrophic scarring, donor sites of the lower extremities are treated much the same as burns are. Depending upon the thickness of the graft taken, these areas usually mature more rapidly than the burns.

Gait abnormalities seen during hospitalization are generally self-limited and occur as a result of pain from burn areas or donor sites. However, children may continue an abnormal gait at home if attention and secondary gain is achieved by this activity either from the family or peer group. Gait should be observed when the patient returns to outpatient clinics and retraining instituted to avoid more serious postural problems.

Burns of the feet may require an alteration of footwear. Foot needs depend upon the location of the burn and residual edema. Many patients wear tennis shoes with or without foam lining until scars become more mature and less sensitive. High top tennis shoes can be used if there is a problem with friction either over the dorsum of the foot or at the calcaneal tendon. Tennis shoes provide a cost-effective, temporary method for dealing with the problems of foot burns while allowing the patient to remain active. Many patients find that after full recovery, they require a larger shoe size than they did prior to the injury.

Some long-term complications of severe lower extremity burns are skin breakdowns due to friction, constant itching and throbbing, and occasional persistent edema formation (Fig. 6-13). Standing is not well-tolerated because of the unpleasant sensations frequently encountered upon assuming an upright position. The patient whose occupation requires long periods of standing may need to be retrained in some other form of employment. Neurological complications have been observed in both burned and unburned lower extremities following severe flame or electrical burn injuries. Lower extremity weakness or paralysis may result from a coincidental spinal cord injury or as a consequence of electrical injury. Henderson et al. and Helm et al. have discussed the presence of peripheral neuropathy of the peroneal nerve following burn injury.[21,22] Damage to this nerve can result in the loss of function, necessitating either temporary or permanent bracing at the ankle.

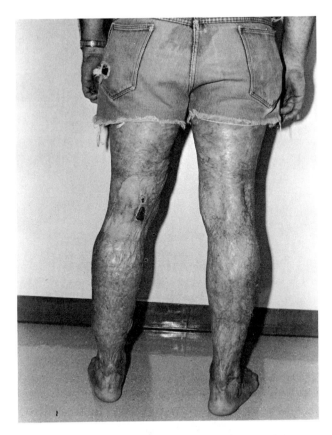

Fig. 6-13. Skin breakdown at popliteal area three years after burn injury. Also note chronic subcutaneous fibrous thickening of the right leg.

BURNS OF THE TRUNK

Sequelae of trunk burns are mainly dependent upon the location and depth of the injury. In full-thickness chest burns, midlateral escharotomies of circumferential trunk eschars may be necessary during the emergent phase to allow for full normal chest excursion. Pain and tight circumferential dressings during the acute phase can also interfere with normal respirations.

Frequent change of position and the use of some form of pressure distribution bed will help prevent pressure sores of the sacrum and scapulae. The head, shoulders, and hips should be aligned properly whether the patient is supine, prone, or on his side. Proper positioning of the trunk can alleviate the need for tedious posture retraining when the patient begins to ambulate.

Following the application of autografts to the posterior trunk, the patient may be required to lie prone for five to seven days. The use of this position should be limited because it interferes with general body flexibility, upper extremity movement, and lung ventilation. Support of the shoulders can help prevent protraction of the shoulders.

Scar contracture of the trunk usually occurs in combination with contractures of the neck and upper or lower extremities. A contracture of the upper chest in continuity with a contracture of the neck and upper extremities can cause protraction of the shoulders and kyphosis. Unilateral trunk burns or circumferential trunk burns of varying depth can lead to functional scoliosis (Fig. 6-14). Pressure garments can aid in minimizing trunk scarring and contracture; however, once apparent, these deformities usually require rapid surgical intervention.

The production of adequate pressure in the shoulder and chest areas may be prevented because of the bridging of the pressure garments over adjacent bony prominences. In these circumstances, foam or elastomer may be added under the pressure garments for additional pressure in the difficult areas.

After healing, restrictive chest scarring may interfere with respiratory function and growth in children. Reconstructive surgical procedures may be needed to allow for contracture release and growth. In a young female with tight chest scarring, re-

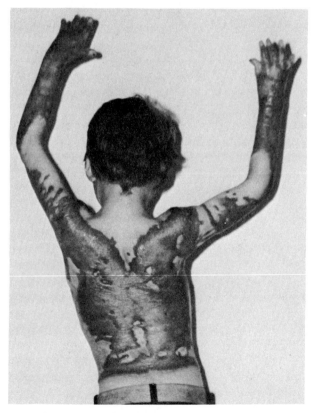

Fig. 6-14. Young patient with functional scoliosis upon movement. Note the presence of thick, unyielding, restricting hypertrophic scarring.

constructive surgical procedures may be needed to allow for normal breast location and development.

MUSCULOSKELETAL PROBLEMS

Heterotopic Calcification

Heterotopic calcification is a complication following burn injury most often found in the elbow joint, but also reported in other major joints in both burned and unburned extremities.[23,24] It occurs late in burn treatment, either near the end of the wound-healing process or after the patient has been discharged from the hospital. Symptoms of heterotopic calcification are increased difficulty in exercise, limitation of range of motion, and pain in the joint. In the elbow, this pain is usually superior to the olecranon process. Roentgenographic examination usually reveals a radiopaque fluffy amorphous mass around the joint (Fig. 6-15).

As calcification can severely limit the range of motion, exercises should continue to prevent fusion of the joint, which may occur with prolonged periods of immobilization. Splinting schedules are adjusted to avoid such prolonged periods of immobilization. Surgical manipulation under anesthesia can be helpful if the patient's condition is recognized early and the patient is experiencing extreme pain and difficulty in range of motion. In the patient with severe pain, limitation of range of motion, or elbow fusion, a surgical procedure can remove the bony block to restore functional range of motion.

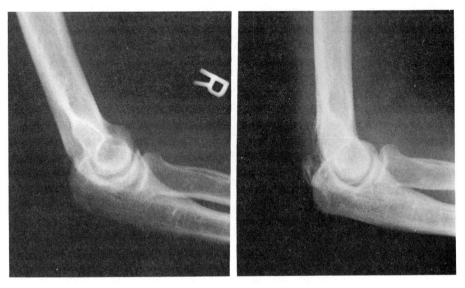

Fig. 6-15. Roentgenograph of elbow showing initial amorphous calcification superior to olecranon and progression of calcification five months later.

Skeletal Fixation

Skeletal fixation can be useful in reducing fractures and providing immobilization after autografts. Positioning must be closely supervised to assure proper alignment. Care should be taken in inserting skeletal fixation devices to avoid damage to underlying structures. Damage to epiphyseal cartilage in children is of particular concern. Proper daily wound care around the pin site is necessary to help prevent osteomyelitis. A common use of skeletal fixation in reconstructive surgical procedures is in alignment of the joints of the fingers.

Fractures and Dislocations

Fractures and dislocations should be anticipated whenever the burn injury is the result of a motor vehicle accident, explosion, electrical burn injury, or other type of violent trauma. When burned skin overlies fracture sites, alterations in treatment are obviously necessary. Surgical procedures normally indicated for fracture reduction may not be possible because of the delicate clinical situation or because of the danger of infection from the surrounding burn wound. In these cases, external splinting devices for skeletal fixation may be utilized to reduce the fracture and at the same time allow exposure of the burn wound for treatment.

Exercise programs should take into consideration the increased metabolic demands of the burn patient with fractures, as well as the increased period of immobilization that is usually necessary. Dislocations are less frequently seen and should be reduced as quickly as possible. Obviously, both fractures and dislocations can limit the positions that the patient can assume while in bed, thus increasing the possibility of contracture, decubiti, and respiratory complications.

Burns of the Perineum

Acute Care Considerations.   Common causes of perineal burn injuries are scalds from hot liquids and bathtub water, flame, and electrical burn injuries. The extent of perineal burn injury may vary from superficial tissue loss to the devastating loss of genitalia and perineal musculature. Because of the natural moist, warm environment of the perineum and the proximity of the wounds to contamination from urine and feces, infection is common in all perineal burns.

Proper wound care during the acute phase should include shaving of all hair around the perineum, thorough daily cleansing, and application of an effective topical antimicrobial. Prompt removal of soiled dressings and linens, cleansing, and reapplication of the topical agent after urination and bowel movements can minimize contamination and help prevent cross-contamination to other sites of burn injury. To prevent such soiling in severe injury, an indwelling urethral catheter can be continued until the wound totally heals. The risk of bladder and kidney infection during long-term catheterization is decreased by positioning the urine collection bag well below the level of the bladder during all activities and by avoiding constriction and clamping of the catheter tubing.

Conservative debridement of the perineal wound is recommended, because

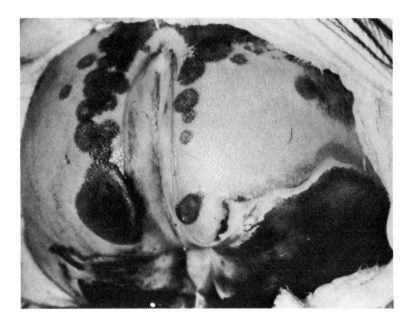

Fig. 6-16.   Perineal wounds must be inspected daily for signs of infection (see text).

structures such as the testes and penis, which may initially appear nonviable, may surprisingly heal and become functional.[25] The wound should be observed daily to detect signs of infection and possible metastatic bacterial lesions, which may indicate infection in other areas of the body (Fig. 6-16). If autografts are necessary, medications can be used to decrease the number and volume of bowel movements, which could cause graft contamination and loss.

In patients with burns of the buttocks, any movement in bed can be limited by pain. It may be helpful in such situations to provide the patient with an overhead trapeze to ease the pain of movement and to allow more independent transfers in and out of bed. Providing smooth dressings and bedding and the use of a padded chair when sitting may also help relieve discomfort. If healed buttock burns continue to be uncomfortable, the patient may want to incorporate foam padding under pressure dressings or under clothing, or use pads while sitting in a chair.

Both the burned and unburned perineum may have complications, such as scrotal and labial edema, decubiti, hemorrhoids, and dermatitis. Scrotal and labial edema during the emergent phase may be severely painful. If the patient can ambulate, a wide based gait may be necessary because of this edema. An explanation to the patient as to the cause and the limited course of such edema should satisfy unexpressed fears of sterility and loss of sexuality.[26]

The patient with perineal burns is at great risk to develop pressure sores over the sacrum and greater trochanters. The patient who is obese, confused, lethargic, or elderly is at even higher risk because of the inability to spontaneously change body positions, decreased skin sensations, or inability to communicate discomfort. Preventive measures include frequent turning, massage of the unburned areas over bony prominences, prompt changes of soiled bedding to avoid skin maceration, and preparation of bed and dressings to avoid wrinkles.

Medical management of hemorrhoids can decrease pain of bowel movements and sitting, leading to improved feelings of well-being. Dermatitis of the perineal and buttock areas can be seen in both children and adults in the acute rehabilitative phases. The etiology of such dermatitis should be determined and treatment instituted as soon as possible.

Rehabilitative Phase Considerations. Skin contractures of the groin and perineum are difficult to prevent. Commercially made elastic panty girdles can control the buttocks, suprapubic, and inner thigh region scarring. Applying foam over healed groin injuries with a figure of eight dressing is sometimes effective in preventing skin contractures. Due to movement and bridging of the garments over the perineum, complete contact with the scar is usually not possible. Using orthotic pressure devices to minimize perineal contractures is generally not practical because of the awkwardness in application and difficulty in maintaining cleanliness of such devices. For young children, cleanliness of garments and orthotics around the perineum can be extremely difficult and can cause parents to discontinue their use because of frustration.

Exercises of pelvic and hip musculature started during the acute phase may not only maintain awareness of muscular function, but also aid in the prevention of decubiti and maintenance of sphincter control. Hip abduction exercises can maintain hip range of motion and aid in stretching of the medial groin and perineal skin. Pelvic exercise after healing can improve muscular awareness and strength and subsequently improve sexual function.

Psychological Considerations. Although the wound is of paramount importance, the psychological effects of burns to the genitalia and perineum cannot be overlooked. Such psychological trauma may be significant and not openly expressed by the patient. Patients have complained of humiliation of having the genitalia unnecessarily exposed during treatment or burn team rounds. The adolescent may be especially vulnerable to such feelings of embarrassment. This anguish can be lessened by providing privacy and appropriate draping of the genitalia whenever possible.

Societal mores and personal feelings about genitalia are integral to the sexuality of a person. All patients with perineal burns should have counseling regarding their sexual functioning. To those patients who have severe burn injury to or loss of genitalia, psychological counseling should begin soon after admission and be continued until the patient can demonstrate a healthy adaptation to such deformity. Reconstructive surgical procedures may prolong the adjustment process. Strictures of the urethra, vagina, or anus may require surgical release to allow normal functioning. With complete loss of genitalia, reconstructive surgical procedures may be helpful in rebuilding genitalia, but the outcome may not be known for many months. Knowledge of the probable outcome of surgical procedures can aid the patient in a realistic adaptation.

REFERENCES

1. Surveyer JA: Smoke inhalation injuries. Heart and Lung 9:825–832, 1980
2. Bendixen HH, Smith GM, Mead J: The pattern of ventilation in young adults. J Appl Physiol 19:195–198, 1964
3. Craven JL, Evans GA, Davenport PJ, Williams RHP: The evaluation of the incentive spirometer in the management of postoperative pulmonary complications. Br J Surg 61:793–797, 1974
4. Whitener DR, Whitener LM, Robertson, KJ, Baxter CR, Pierce AK: Pulmonary function measurements in patients with thermal injury and smoke inhalation. Am Rev Resp Dis 122:731–739, 1980
5. Burns CL, Chylack LT: Thermal burns: the management of thermal burns of the lids and globes. Ann Ophthal 1358–1368, September 1979
6. Rivers EA, Strate RG, Solem LD: The transparent face mask. Am J Occup Ther 33:108–113, 1979
7. Baxter CR: Present concepts in the management of major electrical injury. Surg Clin North Am 50:1401–1418, 1970
8. Feldman AE, MacMillan BG: Burn injury in children: declining need for reconstructive surgery as related to use of neck orthoses. Arch Phys Med Rehabil 61:441–449, 1980
9. Cronin TD: Successful correction of extensive scar contractures of the neck using split skin grafts. Translations of the International Society of Plastic Surgeons (First Congress 1955) Baltimore, Williams & Wilkins, 1957
10. Converse JM: Burn deformities of the face and neck. Surg Clin North Am 47:323–54, 1967
11. Willis B: The use of orthoplast isoprene splints in the treatment of the acutely burned child. Am J Occup Ther 24:187–191, 1970
12. Sinha JK, Khanna NN, Tripathi FM, Bhattacharya V, Chowdhary MD: Electrical burns, a review of 80 cases. Burns 4:261–266
13. Achauer BM, Bartlett RH, Furnas DW, Allyn PA, Wingerson E: Internal fixation in the management of the burned hand. Arch Surg 108:814–820, 1974
14. Alexander JW, MacMillan BG, Martel L, Krummel R: Surgical correction of postburn flexion contractures of the fingers in children. Plast Reconstr Surg 68:218–224, 1981
15. Earle AS, Fratianne RB: Delayed definitive reconstruction of the burned hand: evolution of a program of care. J Trauma 19:149–152, 1979
16. Boswick JA: The management of fresh burns of the hand and deformities resulting from burn injuries. Clin Plast Surg 1:621–631, 1974
17. Whitson TC, Bohn DA: Management of the burned hand. J Trauma 11:606–614, 1971
18. Frank DH, Robson MC: Unusual occurrence of chronic nerve compression syndromes at the wrists of thermally injured patients. Orthop Rev 8:180–183, 1979
19. Fissette J, Onkelux A, Fandi N: Carpal and Guyon tunnel syndromes in burns at the wrist. J Hand Surg 6:13–15, 1981
20. Huang TT, Blackwell SJ, Lewis SR: Ten years of experience in managing patients with burn contractures of axilla, elbow, wrist, and knee joints. Plast Reconstr Surg 61:70–76, 1978
21. Henderson B, Koepke G, Feller I: Peripheral neurological problems among patients with burns. Arch Phys Med Rehab 52:149–151, 1971
22. Helm, PA, Johnson ER, Carlton AM: Peripheral neurological problems in the acute burn patient. Burns 3:123–125

23. Munster AM, Bruck HM, Johns LA, VonPrince K, Kirkman EM, Remig RL: Heterotopic calcification following burns: a prospective study. J Trauma 12:1071–1074, 1973
24. Evans, EB: Orthopedic measures in the treatment of severe burns. J Bone Jt Surg 48A:643–669, 1966
25. McDougal WS, Peterson HD, Pruitt BA, Persky L: The thermally injured perineum. J Urol 121:320–323, 1979
26. Andreasen NJC, Norris HS: Long-term adjustment and adaptation mechanisms in severely burned adults. J Nerv Ment Dis 154:352–362, 1972

7 | Burns in Children

Nancy Newton Hanson

A burn injury at any age level is a tragedy. When a child is involved, the tragedy seems even greater. A child carries with him the hopes of his family and society. He has his whole life ahead of him. When a child is seriously burned, the feelings of guilt, sadness, and needless suffering are sensed by everyone who comes into contact with the child.

The child himself often feels frightened, helpless, lonely, and isolated. He is unable to understand his pain and is frequently unable to understand the rationale for his treatments. His parents often feel they have failed in their role as protector of their child. They usually suffer feelings of guilt and anger, and at times, misdirect it toward the staff.[1] Even the hospital caretakers feel the tragedy. They may be reluctant to cause the child any additional pain associated with therapy, or they may be unsure how to approach and deal with the child.

Special circumstances and concerns always surround the care of a hospitalized child, particularly the burned child. Rehabilitating a burned child is a long, difficult, and challenging undertaking. This chapter will be devoted to this unique and very rewarding challenge.

The chapter will begin by addressing some of the special problems surrounding the treatment of burned children and by offering some suggestions on how to manage these problems. The chapter will also offer the therapist some suggestions on how to approach children and will suggest some ways in which a burn facility as a whole can help a child cope with his injury. Hopefully, with a greater understanding of the burned child, the therapist will be better equipped to accept this special rehabilitative challenge.

TECHNICAL PROBLEMS IN REHABILITATION

The general principles and objectives of pediatric burn care are similar to those of adult burn care. Wounds must be dressed and kept clean. Affected joints must be

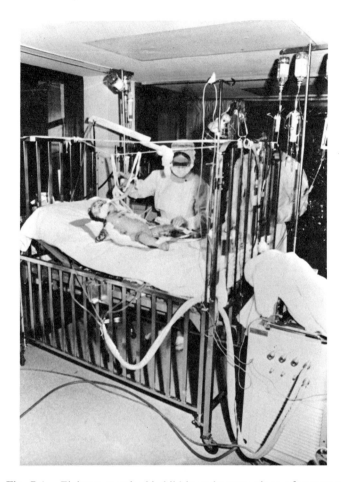

Fig. 7-1.   Eighteen-month-old child in early acute phase of recovery.

positioned and splinted to reduce contracture formation (see Ch. 3).[2] Exercise programs should be well-planned and conscientiously carried out in order to reduce joint stiffness, and functional activities must be stressed (see Ch. 4).[3] Rehabilitation goals in children are much the same as those in adults. The significant difference between children and adults is in the practical application of the basic rehabilitation techniques and in the method of approach.

Evaluation of the Burn

An initial evaluation of the burned child should be made as soon as possible after admission.[4] The depth of burns in children is notoriously difficult to assess initially, and frequently must be made retrospectively.[5] This is particularly true of second-degree burns. In some children, a superficial second-degree burn may initially appear much deeper. Conversely, a deep second- or third-degree burn in a very small child may have the pink or mottled red appearance of a superficial to medium depth burn, only to declare its full thickness later on. Sensation to pinprick may also be hard to test in an uncooperative child.

Thus, when evaluating the depth of the burns in a child, it helps to consider the etiology of the burn.[5] Flame burns, for example, are usually deep, whereas hot water scalds are frequently, but not always, more superficial. Burns associated with flammable liquids, such as gasoline, also tend to be deep. In general, it is probably best either to delay estimation of depth until the burns declare themselves several days later or to be conservative and estimate on the deeper side.[5]

Once the child has been evaluated, a rehabilitation program should be carefully planned. It is helpful if this plan can be formulated and initiated as early as possible.[6] Although a child may dislike portions or all of his therapy, it is usually easier for him to adapt if it is begun soon after admission and carried through conscientiously. He thus learns that a particular splint or exercise regime is part of the hospital therapy and he usually accepts it more graciously than if it were introduced later on. It is also obvious that if physical and occupational therapy are begun early, less rehabilitation problems are likely to develop.[7]

Positioning and Splinting

Adequate positioning and splinting of the burned child can be a tremendous challenge. Positioning may be difficult because parents, and sometimes hospital personnel, may feel sorry for the child, whose movement is restrained by dressings and splints. It is often feared that a child's physical and/or emotional development may suffer if he is not free to move around. In this situation, it is helpful to point out that the burn injury is serious and must assume a certain amount of priority. After healing, almost all children will rapidly make up for temporary setbacks in their physical and psychological development.[8]

It is well-known that proper positioning and splinting may greatly reduce the development of contractures;[9] thus, in the long run there will actually be less interference with the child's development than if contractures were allowed to develop. Once established, contractures often require future hospitalizations and surgical procedures for correction. Movement must again be restrained postoperatively, and the repeated hospital admissions are stressful to both child and family.

It thus becomes clear that one must resist the tendency to feel misguided sympathy for the child and one must maintain a certain amount of firmness in insisting that the positioning program be followed. Often, this is not easy. Sometimes there is an emotional barrier that the therapist must overcome by convincing himself that he is doing the right thing. It is useful for the therapist to keep the long-term goals clearly in mind and not focus too much on the child's present unhappiness and tears. It is also imperative that the necessity for positioning and splinting be explained to both the child and parents. Many parents and older children are likely to be more cooperative if they truly understand the objectives of the splinting program and the long-term consequences of inadequate splinting.

It is important that all members of the burn team understand the program and, by working together, present a unified front to child and family. A therapist will be

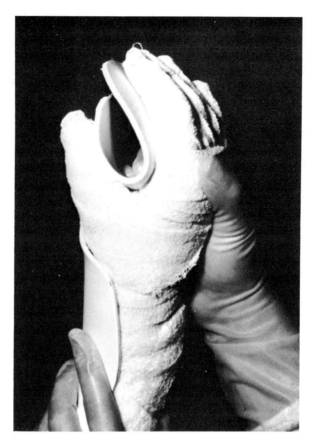

Fig. 7-2.   Proper positioning and splinting of burned hand of child. Note that MCP joints are at approximately 70°, PIP and DIP joints in full extension, and thumb in abducted, opposed position.

much more successful in achieving proper positioning if he or she has the support and understanding of all staff that come into contact with the child.[6] It is also easier for the child to accept the positioning program if the nurses, doctors, and physical and occupational therapists are all consistent in their approach.

Proper positioning and splinting is difficult with children because they are physically active and almost constantly in motion. Because of this tendency of children to move about, the therapist may find it almost impossible to keep them in certain positions. This problem can be alleviated somewhat by making sure that splints are well-contoured, padded if necessary, and firmly secured to the patient. An effort should be made to involve the nonsplinted parts of the child's body with outside activities whenever feasible; for example, using the nonsplinted hand to play a game. If that is not possible, selecting a game that the child can play even with a handsplint

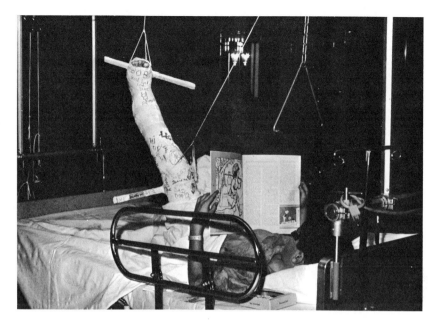

Fig. 7-3. Distraction helps the child focus his attention away from himself.

in place is often successful. Distraction, whenever possible, is an extremely useful tool, as it allows the child to focus his attentions on things other than his own discomfort and splints. Some children draw support from the knowledge that other children must also wear splints and that they "are all in the same boat."[10]

A child who is positioned in bed with his neck in extension may have great difficulty seeing what is going on. Every effort should be made to turn the child's bed so that he can see the activities that are taking place within the room. If the child is not being isolated, his entire bed can be brought to a playroom or to a place where he can interact with other children.

Splinting may be difficult in children because of the small sizes involved. This is particularly true in very young children. Fabrication of a well-fitting hand splint for a one- or two-year-old child is truly a challenge. The distance between the child's metacarpophalangeal joints and his interphalangeal joints may be only a few millimeters. Therefore, it is almost impossible to achieve a perfect fit initially. A therapist must accept the fact that such a splint will probably require frequent alterations. These alterations also allow for the dissipation of initial edema formation, and for changes in range of motion.[11]

These small splints are easier to keep in place if secured with small gauze wraps; for example, two-inch-wide gauze will often work better than three- or four-inch-wide gauze. Well-placed straps can also help to secure small splints. Sometimes a combination of both gauze wraps and strapping may be necessary to hold a splint in the proper position.

Another problem with splinting in children is the tendnecy to leave them off too long, under the pretext that the child is exercising or using his hands. Naturally, if the child is truly using the extremity in some type of purposeful functional activity, then it is quite desirable to leave the splints off to encourage this activity.[6] This type of functional activity is the ultimate goal of our therapeutic techniques. However, it may be necessary to take a very close look at exactly what the child is really doing during these unsplinted periods. If he is merely moving a toy around by pushing it with the palm of his hand, or if he is taking a three-hour afternoon nap with his knees unsplinted and flexed, it may be better to limit the unsplinted periods and to supervise more closely the child's activities during those times. This is particularly true for children with deep dermal or full-thickness burns, who tend to form contractures quickly.

On the opposite end of the spectrum, a therapist must also be careful not to over immobilize a patient. Patients with superficial burns do not form contractures. To splint a child with such burns may cause unnecessary discomfort and may indeed be harmful. There is a tremendous amount of individual variation among patients, and some do not tend to stiffen as quickly as others. Oversplinting in such patients will only cuase increased frustration to both patient and therapist. These children may be left unsplinted for long periods, or perhaps left completely unsplinted. However, they must be reassessed frequently to ensure that they are not losing range of motion. If their functional ability and range of motion remain adequate, then these lucky patients may do quite well on an exercise program alone.

Postoperative positioning of the newly grafted burn patient may be quite difficult. Immobilization during this time is crucial, since excessive movements may jeopardize the healing of skin grafts. Children may be immobilized after surgery by using bulky dressings, splints, or casts.[3] K-wire traction is sometimes used because it helps to suspend and elevate an extremity and reduce any tendency to rub the affected area on the bed sheets.[6,12] Although postoperative medication is not desirable, in some cases a particularly active child may require it for a few days to reduce activity to an acceptable level. This must be done with careful monitoring to prevent pneumonia, pressure sores, and other sequelae of inactivity.

Whatever method of immobilization is used, it is helpful for the therapist to discuss this postoperative plan thoroughly with other members of the burn team prior to the operative procedure. This allows the burn team a chance to formulate a mutually agreeable plan in advance of the anticipated procedure. Any necessary splints can be prepared ahead of time or in the operating room and, if required, the patient's bed can be equipped with the proper traction equipment.

Preparing a postoperative treatment plan is also useful because it then becomes possible to discuss this plan preoperatively with the patient. Most children fear surgery, but some of their anxiety can be relieved if they understand why their arm will be suspended from a Balkan frame or in a particular splint when they awaken. Since their cooperation after surgery is so important, several preoperative teaching-information sessions are highly beneficial. These sessions can also serve to provide the child with information concerning donor sites, skin grafts, and healing. Obviously, the amount of information given and abosrbed will depend upon the child's age, his general inquisitiveness, and upon what is deemed appropriate at the time.

Exercise Therapy

Exercise therapy has long been recognized as an important tool in the maintenance of joint range of motion.[4] However, when dealing with children, the execution of an effective exercise program is complicated by the inability of some children, especially younger ones, to understand the importance of their therapy.[3] Small children tend to think in terms of the present time. They are unable to conceptualize that if they work hard on their therapy now, they will be rewarded by successful rehabilitation in the future. They are mainly concerned with the pain and discomfort they feel at the moment. This failure to understand long-term consequences can lead to what may appear, to the unsympathetic adult, as uncooperativeness and resistance.[13] Some children can become so difficult that they actually exhibit detrimental behavior, such as adamant refusal to exercise or destruction of their skin grafts.[13] These children are a particularly difficult challenge and must be understood and handled with great care.

In contrast, some children, particularly older ones, can be quite rational about the necessity for exercise. For these children, it is quite important to take the time to carefully explain the importance of exercising.[14] The explanations should be simple, and the benefits of the child's cooperation should be explained in terms that are significant to the child. Approaches such as "when you are healed" and "when you are able to use your hand, you'll be able to go home" should be used. It helps if the

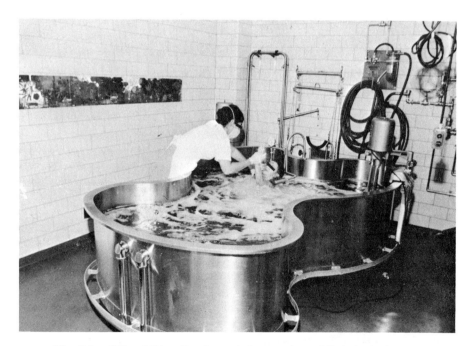

Fig. 7-4. Older child performing resistive exercises while in hydrotherapy.

child is aware of his general treatment plan and his progress, and realizes that his cooperation may speed up his recovery.

Sometimes children can be lured into an exercise program by making the sessions into games or by making the activities fun.[3] This requires a certain degree of imagination on the part of the therapist. It is usually helpful to talk to the child or his parents to find out the child's particular play interests, such as building blocks, making models, playing ball, and so on. If the child's individual interests are considered when planning his exercise program, he may be much more cooperative.

Another possible way to induce a child's cooperation is to offer him choices in therapy.[14] When doing this, the therapist must be careful to choose alternatives that represent desirable results. This approach is successful because it allows the child to have some control over the situation, and more importantly, to have his choice considered.[14] In this way the child may have some choice about the *way* he does his exercises, but he is *not* given a choice as to whether or not he will do his exercises.

In general, it is helpful to be firm and consistent with children.[3] If a child is allowed to have a day off from his exercises, he or she may try to get away without performing his exercises on the following day. The most successful therapist is one who can remain cheerful but also consistent about important matters such as exercise therapy.

Ambulation

Postoperative ambulation of the child with full-thickness burns of the lower extremities is usually begun about ten days after skin grafting. This period will vary somewhat among individual patients and burn centers. If a child has partial-thickness superficial leg burns, he may be allowed to ambulate throughout his hospitalization. In either case, Ace bandages are almost always indicated and may be applied over gauze leg dressings.[6] Ace wraps will help to reduce oozing and bleeding from any open wounds. They also reduce venous pooling and help to eliminate the tendency for blisters to form in newly healed skin grafts.[6] Between periods of walking, the child should sit or rest with his legs elevated; this will reduce edema formation and the tendency to form flexion contractures at the knee.

For many children, ambulation is something to look forward to. To them, ambulation represents a change for the better, which indeed it is. It represents a step towards normalcy; and the children may be so excited to try walking that the therapist must be sure that they do not exhaust themselves on the first day of ambulation or that in their enthusiasm, they injure themselves.

Some children, however, may fear ambulation. These apprehensive children sometimes feel that they have been at bedrest so long that they simply will not be able to walk. They may become very fearful and may resist attempts to walk or stand. This child needs a lot of patient encouragement. He needs to be assured that he will not be left alone and that he will not fall. This child needs firm physical support from at least one person (preferably two people if the child is older or is extremely apprehensive). After initial attempts at ambulation, he needs to be praised for his efforts and reassured that it may take awhile before he will be able to walk smoothly and independently, but be reassured that he will.

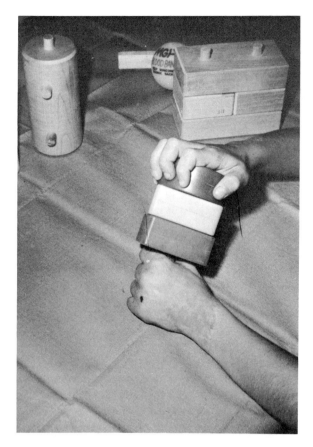

Fig. 7-5. Five-year-old boy with healed skin grafts on the dorsum of the left hand. He enjoyed exercising with blocks.

Scarring and Pressure Therapy

Unfortunately, scarring can be a very real problem in children.[6] Healing of deep dermal or full-thickness burns often leads to thick, red, inelastic hypertrophic scars.[15] As with adults, these scars can be improved by the use of pressure wraps of garments; however, the use of pressure on children presents some special problems.[15]

One problem, unique to children, is that they grow quickly, particularly younger children. This means that custom-fitted pressure garments will need to be replaced frequently. A therapist should check these patients to be sure that the garments fit properly. Sometimes children gain or lose weight after their discharge from the hospital, and this is another reason to schedule checkups in order to assess proper fit. It is usually best to order two sets of garments, so that one can be in the wash while the other is being worn. When elastic wraps are used (e.g., on the arms and legs), it is somewhat easier to accommodate for growth and weight changes.

Sweating and itching can also be a problem.[15] Although itching can occur without exercise, the high activity level of most children causes them to become warm and sweat beneath their pressure garments, resulting in uncomfortableness and itching. In this case, it is helpful to remove the garment, wash the skin, and replace the garment with a clean, dry one. Skin that is well-lubricated with cream tends to itch less; however, one must be careful not to apply a pressure garment until the cream has had a chance to be absorbed by the skin. In severe cases of itching, medication may be of limited use.

One of the most difficult problems surrounding scar-pressure therapy within the pediatric population is lack of cooperation. There is no simple solution to this problem. Perhaps the best way to encourage participation in pressure regimes is to be sure that the parents and the child, if he is old enough, are well-informed about the long-term cosmetic results of adequate pressure on the scars. Sometimes a discussion with another burn patient is helpful, particularly if the other patient was conscientious about his pressure therapy and his scars have become pale, flattened, and mature.

Pressure therapy is usually maintained until the particular scars involved have matured (i.e., they are no longer red, raised, and itchy, and no longer blanch with pressure).[15] For some patients in some locations, scar maturation may occur as early as six months after injury, whereas in other patients in other locations, it may take one and a half years before the scars become pale and flat in appearance.[15] It is often difficult for patients to maintain their pressure program over such a long period of time, and frequent encouragement may be necessary.

Posthospital Care

Posthospital care also presents difficult problems.[3] Many children and their families feel that when the child is discharged he is "all well," and they find it hard to understand that splinting, exercise, and pressure therapy may be necessary for several more months.[16] Many people have difficulty accepting the long-term process of scar maturation and contracture.

When a burned child approaches discharge, it is very important for the burn team members to plan for the child's posthospital care. It is crucial that the child's family understand the daily care that will be required at home.[4] During the patient's last week of hospitalization, it is helpful if the family can make frequent visits to the hospital so that therapists, doctors, and nurses can carefully explain the care necessary after discharge. This usually consists of instructions concerning dressing changes, skin care, medications, splinting, exercise programs, and the use of pressure garments. There may be a lot of technical-medical information for a parent to absorb, and it is best if the family has several days to ask questions, discuss treatments, and watch demonstrations.

Some centers have found it helpful to create discharge manuals to be reviewed with family members prior to discharge. In this way parents have a chance to absorb written material and to practice some of the child's care under medical supervision before the discharge actually takes place. Thus, when they arrive home with the child, they will feel more confident about their ability to carry out the required therapy. It is also helpful if the entire home program is written in simple language so that a parent can easily refer to the written program whenever in doubt.[3]

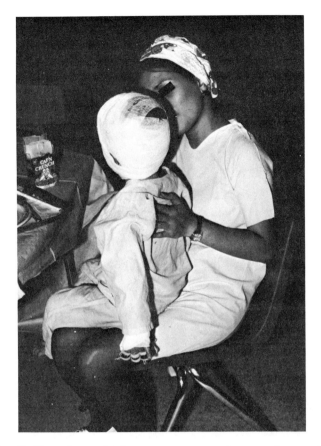

Fig. 7-6. Staff member explaining a treatment procedure to a six-year-old child.

Perhaps the most difficult problem that a therapist faces during posthospital care is the tendency for children to manipulate their parents and thereby fail to carry out their prescribed home programs. This is particularly true if the parents feel guilty about the burn incident. Some children take advantage of feelings of guilt or sympathy and will resist therapy at home, even if they were cooperative while in the hospital. In most cases it is desirable for the burned child to return to the burn facility for outpatient treatments and follow-up care.[3] Frequent checkups will allow the hospital staff to monitor the child's progress, see if the program is being followed, and alter the treatments when necessary. The checkups also enable the staff to detect any problems that may develop and to change therapy courses as necessary.

If the family does not live near the primary care facility, local follow-up care can be arranged.[3] In all cases, however, it is important that the family be encouraged to contact the hospital whenever they have serious concerns or questions. With open communication, the development of subsequent problems can be minimized.

GENERAL PROBLEMS IN REHABILITATION

Pain is one of the most difficult problems to deal with following a burn injury. Pain, however, is a very personal and subjective experience.[17] The actual physical phenomenon of pain is influenced by the patient's mental attitude, his environment, and his upbringing. Pain, or expressions of pain, are therefore variable among different patients.[17]

Pain in a burned child is frequently complicated by the child's fears and anxieties. For example, a child may become very anxious and begin to scream frantically when a therapist asks him to do certain exercises. This is often partly because the child does not know where the therapist will touch him, or how much, if at all, the exercise will actually hurt. Thus, fearing the worst, the child cries and becomes resistant at the very prospect of being moved or touched.[18]

It is very difficult to generalize about how to deal with a burned child's pain. The actual physical aspect of the pain is very real and should be respected. The anxiety associated with the pain may often be relieved by securing the trust and confidence of the patient. This can be done by being straightforward and honest. It helps if the therapist takes some extra time to explain in a simple but detailed way what he will and will not do. It also helps if the therapist can appear as a calm, kind, and caring person who will try to minimize the amount of pain that tte treatment will cause. A therapist should try to remain creative and to keep an open mind about alternative and perhaps less painful ways to achieve the same end. However, a certain amount of pain will probably always be present in a therapy session, and the child should be allowed to express this pain. These expressions, such as crying and screaming, are phenomena that the therapist must personally learn to deal with if he or she is to be effective as a rehabilitation specialist. This author must personally admit that even after nine years of working with children, the sound of a child screaming in pain is still a disturbing and upsetting experience.

In order to tolerate the crying, it may be useful for the therapist to try to look toward the future and try to imagine the child after his rehabilitation is complete. This type of concentration on the long-term goals will help the therapist to deal with the cries of pain in the present and will help to keep the therapeutic objectives in mind.

Experienced therapists and other health care providers have learned to identify the different cries of children in a hospital.[19] This ability allows a therapist to let certain cries, usually the ones not associated with pain, to pass almost unnoticed. This is a protective mechanism that pediatric workers often adopt, and does not necessarily reflect a hardening of the feelings.[19]

As a therapist gains experience, he or she must develop personal ways of coping with the pain that is ever present in burn centers. Individual coping measures vary greatly between professionals on the burn ward. Sometimes, discussions with other burn team members can help in this personal adjustment.

Another problem that a therapist faces is eliciting the motivation of a child.[3] Surely the best possible results will occur in a patient who is motivated toward his own rehabilitation. Securing that motivation, however, is not always easy. It is useful if the therapist spends some time talking with his young patient and discussing the goals of the therapy. If possible, the therapist should try to get the child involved in his own treatments. If the child makes progress or trys hard to cooperate, he should be lavishly praised. A little positive feedback can often go a long way toward stimulating a child to become involved in his care. Sometimes a small reward may be in order, such as a lollipop, a comic book, or staying with the child after the treatment to read a story.

Another general problem in pediatric burns is that patients often develop tremendous feeling of isolation. A child is part of his family and his community, and when removed from these familiar surroundings, he will naturally feel lonely.[20] He is probably suffering the worst hurt in his life and is also being separated from his parents. These feelings are magnified when the patient is physically isolated within the hospital for infection control purposes. To best deal with this problem, all the members of the burn team should visit the child frequently and make an effort to encourage the child's family to visit. A window in the child's room helps the child feel a little less imprisoned. Mechanisms for communication, such as call buttons and telephones, make the child feel as though he can get in touch with the world when he begins to feel lonely or isolated.

APPROACHING THE BURNED CHILD

Every once in a while there is a child that is particularly resistant to therapy. For this type of child, patience, explanations, and efforts to make therapy more pleasant do

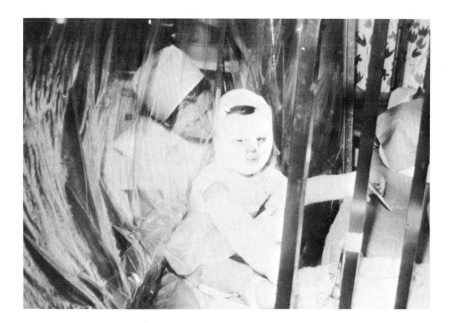

Fig. 7-7. Two-year-old child resisting isolation.

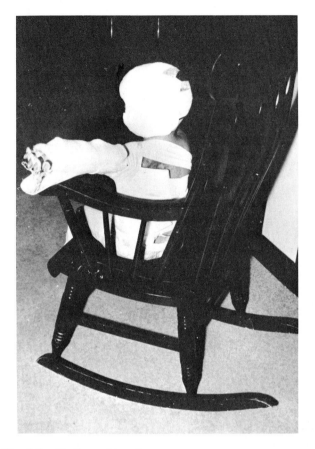

Fig. 7-8. Feelings of loneliness and isolation are inevitable.

not seem to help much. The child may be very skeptical of all hospital workers. Occasionally the therapist can achieve some success by using proper timing; for example, by trying, if possible, not to approach the patient after a painful dressing change or debridement session. In some cases, the physician may feel that medication is in order. This may help to get the child through the most difficult part of his therapy session. When all else fails, the therapist must remain persistent and maintain a mental attitude of "not giving up." It helps to keep in mind that the total healing process is long and complicated, and that, more than ever before, children are surviving after larger and more serious burns.[10] Therefore, the likelihood of treating difficult children is increased.

Although most therapists have developed their own personal style of meeting and dealing with patients, some therapists are reluctant and intimidated at the prospect of approaching a burned child. The therapist's approach is important and it often influences how the child reacts to his total treatment. It is helpful if the therapist begins with a certain amount of confidence in himself and in the importance of the child's therapy program. Children can be very perceptive and can often sense from their therapist the importance of their rehabilitation sessions.

A healthy patient-therapist relationship should be based upon trust.[17] Once an atmosphere of trust is developed between the child and his therapist, the possibility for successful rehabilitation is greatly enhanced. In order to develop this type of relationship, the therapist must strive to be honest with the patient. This means that the child can always rely on the therapist to answer questions honestly and in a simple, straightforward manner. This is especially true of the classic question, "will it hurt"? Whenever possible, this honesty should be combined with a positive attitude. For example, "the first few times that we get you up to walk, it will be difficult, but after a while you will get better at it; and, the sooner that you are able to walk, the sooner you will be able to go home."

It is helpful if the therapist can try to spend time with the patient and to try not to appear too rushed. This may be difficult in a busy setting, but it is useful to remember that a hurried therapist tends to make an anxious child. A therapist who takes extra time to explain treatments or just to talk to a new patient will usually be rewarded in the long run, because the child tends to relax and sense what is expected of him. This usually means that the future treatments will go more smoothly and quickly.

Unfortunately, some children will be very difficult. With these patients, one must remain persistent. They will eventually realize that the therapist will not give in, no matter how much they fuss; and most of these children will give up this fussing when they discover that it is not productive. It is difficult to generalize about

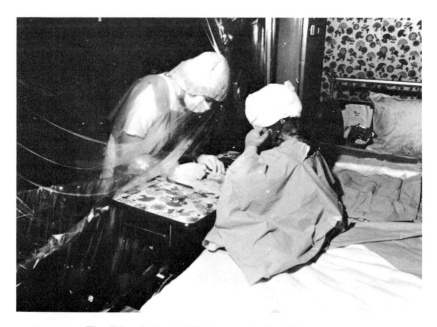

Fig. 7-9. Isolated child "crayoning" with her nurse.

how to approach a burned child because all children all different, and the therapist's approach must be flexible enough to meet the needs of each patient. In general, the therapist should try to remain encouraging and kind to the child, while at the same time be consistently firm about the things that are really important.

SUGGESTIONS FOR DEALING WITH THE SPECIAL PROBLEMS OF THE BURNED CHILD

Successful rehabilitation of a burned child is more likely to be achieved if the child is seen as a whole person with many needs.[20] Most children will require some support during the traumatic ordeal of healing from an injury and in dealing with a hospitalization.[1]

Frequently, psychological support is indicated. In many cases, a sensitive psychiatric nurse or social worker can help a child tremendously. This person can often be a welcome visitor for a child because she does not represent a painful threat. Many hospitals have social workers who regularly visit the patients within the burn unit, and who can also provide a listening ear for a child's questions and problems.[1] Most hospitals also have psychologists or psychiatrists who are available on a consultation basis to help with more difficult or troubled patients.

Another way in which the hospital can help a burned child is by providing an opportunity for the child to relate with his peers.[21] This can be done formally by involving the child in organized peer group sessions with former burn patients. In this manner, successful veterans can help the child by discussing how they dealt with problems such as name calling or staring.[21] Sometimes this type of peer interaction can be achieved informally by providing opportunities for burned children to relate to one another while they are in the hospital setting.

The burn unit or hospital can also help a child by making an effort to provide some time for recreation. Many pediatric settings have playrooms, which are set aside purely for the purpose of recreation. However, where space is limited, such as in a burn center, a special corner will suffice as a play area. If the child is isolated in a room by himself, it is still important to set aside some time for play, and to bring autoclaved toys into the child's room. If feasible, a recreational therapist should see the child, but if this is not possible, parents and well-selected volunteers should be encouraged to visit and play with the child.

It is also important for the burn unit staff to remember that the children of various ages have different needs.[20] Small children need the company of their families and bright, colorful toys. Small children also respond to cuddling and should be held or handled frequently if possible. Adolescents and teenagers often need interaction with others in their own age group. They need privacy and they like records and music. They also need the company of their families, but they may not be willing to admit it. They may resent being treated in the same manner as younger children.

The burn team staff can also help the burned child by providing some type of support system for that child's family.[1] Some authorities feel that the single most important factor in the social recovery of a burned child is a loving and accepting family. Family members may, however, undergo tremendous guilt and agony over a

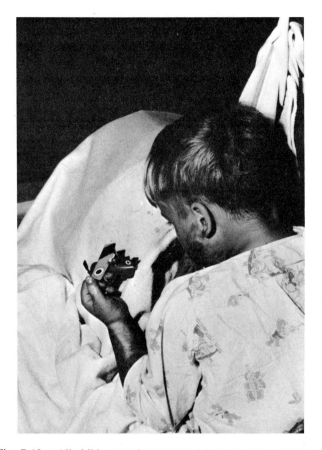

Fig. 7-10. All children need toys, especially the hospitalized child.

burn accident. They will be much better equipped to help and support their child if they themselves can have some help in dealing with these negative feelings. Parents can often be supported by the social worker assigned to the child's case, or by parent group sessions.[1] It is worthwhile to note that parents are usually more relaxed and comfortable when the therapist and nurses take time to discuss their child's treatments and progress on a regular basis.

In addition, the hospital can help the child by trying to smooth the child's eventual return to school.[22] This reentry into school after a burn injury can be a much-feared event. The hospital can be of assistance by staying in contact with the child's school while he is hospitalized and by encouraging the child's teacher and classmates to correspond with the child.[22] This helps the child to feel that he has friends and that he has not been forgotten while he is in the hospital. Letters or tape-recorded messages are useful for this purpose. Sometimes the child's teacher can be encouraged to visit him during his hospitalization.[23] The teacher may be useful in preparing the classroom for the return of the child and for setting an atmosphere of acceptance within the classroom.[23] This can be a tremendous help to a frightened child. Hope-

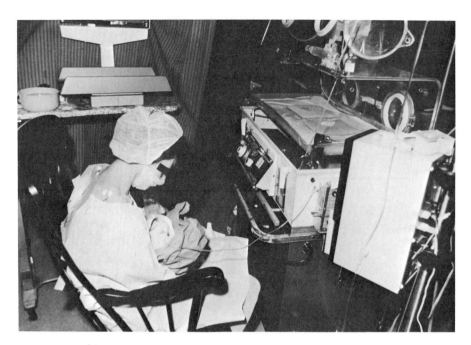

Fig. 7-11. Even the smallest patients are receptive to tenderness.

fully, the child can be encouraged to return to school as soon as he is medically ready. It is usually a little easier if the child and his family do not postpone this important event by seeking private tutors. The longer the event is postponed, the more difficult it often becomes.[23]

SUMMARY AND CONCLUSIONS

For the therapist, physical rehabilitation of the burned child is a long struggle— initially against life threatening forces and eventually against scar formation and scar contracture. This struggle is complicated by the numerous psychological ramifications that accompany a burn injury.

Children go through definite stages during their struggle to recover. Initially, the child often fears the pain of his dressing changes and the sight of his wounds. He may also fear death or may fear that he will not be able to walk again. As the healing progresses and functional ability improves the child may begin to worry about his appearance, rejection, and future in general. An astute therapist should try to remain aware of the child's thoughts and feelings as the child progresses, and should remember that each child is a little different in his pattern of adjustment.

Physical rehabilitation should be individualized to meet each child's physical goals, while also considering his emotional state.[4] Throughout the recovery process, the child's progress should be monitored and the therapy program altered to address the child's current problems and needs.[24] Whenever possible, the therapist should try to stimulate motivation.

When dealing with children, the following five suggestions are offered: (1) be honest; (2) explain the treatment procedures ahead of time; (3) be firm and consistent, yet understanding; (4) try to have some fun with the child; and (5) let the child know that you care for him. Successful rehabilitation of a burned child is probably one of the greatest challenges that a therapist can undertake. Both therapist and patient will have moments of frustration. The recovery process is long and often complicated, but the reward of seeing a child who has been successfully rehabilitated after a burn injury is extremely gratifying. It is well worth the hard work. If the therapist can apply the basic rehabilitation principles that relate to all burn injuries, while at the same time take into consideration the special problems of children, the challenge of rehabilitating the burned child can be more successfully met.

REFERENCES

1. Cahners SS, Bernstein, NR: Rehabilitating families with burned children. Scand J Plast Reconstr Surg 13:173–175, 1979
2. Evans EB, Larson DL, Yates S: Joint function in patients with severe burns. Mod Med of Aus 14:67–69, 1969
3. Newton N, Bubenickova M: Rehabilitation of the autografted hand in children with burns. Phys Ther 57:1383–1387, 1977
4. Jaeger MA: Maintenance of function of the burn patient. Phys Ther 52:627–633, 1972
5. Fichandler BC, Heinrich JJ, Robson MC: Outpatient management of burns. The PA Journal Fall:30–34, 1974
6. Baebel S, Bulkley AL, Shuck JM: Physical therapy for burned patients—low budget effectiveness. Phys Ther 53:1289–1293, 1973
7. MacMillian B: Burns in children. Clin Plas Surg 1:633–643, 1974
8. McCall RB: Milestones of growth. In: Infants. Cambridge, Harvard University Press, 1979
9. Willis B: The use of orthoplast isoprene splints in the treatment of the acutely burned child. Am J of Occup Ther 24:187–191, 1970
10. Bernstein NR: Emotional problems of the facially burned and disfigured. Boston, Little Brown and Company, 1976
11. Lavore JS, Marshall JH: Expedient splinting of the burned patient. Phys Ther 52:1036–1042, 1972
12. Larson DL, Abston S, Goldman A: The burned child. Tex Med 67:58–67, 1971
13. Currier LM, Torgerson FG, Friz BR: The physical therapist and the management of emotional reactions to physical disability. Phys Ther 40:17–29, 1960
14. Blake FG: Immobilized youth—a rationale for supportive nursing intervention. Am J Nurs 69:2364–2369, 1969
15. Larson DL, Abston S, Evans EB, Dobrkovsky M, Linares HA: Techniques for decreasing scar formation and contractures in the burned patient. J Trauma 11:807–823, 1971
16. Seeger SJ, Schaefer AA: The treatment of burns. Physiotherapy Rev 14:174–176, 1934
17. Hislip HJ: Pain and exercise. J Am Phys Ther Assoc 40:98–105, 1960
18. Holland EJ: The role of physical therapy in the rehabilitation of burn patients. Phys Ther Rev 32:244–246, 1952
19. Nelson A: How can you stand the crying. Am J Nurs 70:66–69, 1970

20. Arrington BS: The pediatric patient. J Am Phys Ther Assoc 42:168–171, 1962
21. Guggenheim FG, O'Hara S: Peer counseling in a general hospital. Am J Psychiatry 133:1197–1199, 1976
22. deWet B, Cwyes S, Davies MQ, Vander Riet R: Some aspects of post treatment adjustment in severely burned children. Burns 5:321–325, 1979
23. Cahners S: A strong hospital—school liason: a necessity for good rehabilitation planning for disfigured children. Scand J Plas Reconstr Surg 13:167–181, 1979
24. Prior MM, Jaeger L: Physical therapy in the treatment of burns. Phys Ther Rev 32:510–513, 1952

8 | Posthospitalization Care

Julianne W. Howell

"Returning to society as a productive individual is a difficult task
for many burn patients. Progress in the rehabilitation program depends
on the patient's personal commitment; as well as the health team's ability to provide firm and intelligent guidance throughout the lengthy rehabilitation phase of care."[1]

Rehabilitation for the burn victim should commence at the time of injury and
may extend to an average of one to two years beyond the initial hospitalization.[2]
Although the patient, family, and individual burn team members may have been
thoroughly informed of the essentials of burn care, the patient and individual burn
team member will likely encounter problems that they cannot manage themselves.
Therefore, coordination of the burn team effort is essential to bridge the often difficult gap between hospitalization and postdischarge care.

The objective of the following discussion is to elaborate on the physical therapist's role in posthospitalization care of the burn patient. This will include theories
of hypertrophic scarring, contractures, and exercise. Application and evaluation of
the concepts of exercise, splinting, positioning, and pressure in the latter stages of
care will be overviewed. Rationale will be offered for the use of modalities to aug-
ment the therapeutic program. Numerous problems unique to the burn patient are
supplemented with suggestions for clinical intervention.

THEORY OF HYPERTROPHIC SCARRING AND CONTRACTURES

Hypertrophic scarring and contracture is more likely to occur if the initial burn injury
has gone to or beyond the level of the reticular dermis (deep partial-thickness or deep

second-degree burn). "Healing of the deep wound results in the replacement of normal integument with a mass of metabolically highly active tissues lacking the normal architecture of the skin."[3]

Several theories have been formulated to explain the processes involved in burn scar hypertrophy and contracture. The most widely-accepted theory postulates that there are several different processes at work in the healing and the healed wound. These processes include the following:

1. Mass production of large amounts of fused highly disorganized collagen.
2. Replacement of the normal dermal elastic ground substance with inelastic chondroitin sulfate A.
3. Involuntary contraction of myofibroblasts, a recently discovered cell normally found in open healing wounds and having some elements of smooth muscle.
4. The inflammatory response elicited by mast cells.
5. Increased vascularity and localized lymphedema.
6. Compaction of the connective tissue by voluntary contraction of the skeletal muscle.

The bonds between the twisted collagen and firm inelastic ground substance, coupled with the simultaneous contraction of the myofibroblasts, contribute to the "heaped up" appearance of the hypertrophic scar. In addition, the frequent use of underlying voluntary skeletal muscle reinforces the compaction of the collagen. To minimize the powerful effects of the myofibroblasts and underlying muscle, these processes must be met by equal counterforces.

The intensity and duration of the vascular response provides a visible clue to the likelihood of hypertrophic scarring and contracture formation.[2] The hyperemia of the scar tissue signifies ongoing change within the closed wound. As long as this clinical characteristic persists, scar maturation has not been completed, and hypertrophy is a possibility.

This active phase gradually diminishes and will usually be completed in an average of one and a half to two years postburn. If appropriate measures are instituted during this active period, the scar tissue loses its redness and softens. Linares has shown that "pressure induces loosening of collagen bundles and encourages parallel orientation of the collagen bundles to the skin surface with the disappearance of the dermal nodules."[3] With the application of pressure, there is a coincident restructuring of the collagen mass and a decrease in vascularity and cellularity.

To inhibit the natural sequelae of the burn injury and to insure the most favorable postinjury result, programs should be instituted that include both counterforces and significant pressures (Fig. 8-1).

PRINCIPLES OF PRESSURE AND INCREASING RANGE OF MOTION

Pressure

Larson has shown that at least 25 mmHg pressure must be achieved to provide histologically and clinically significant pressure.[4] Even as much as 40 mmHg pres-

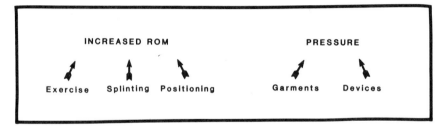

INCREASED ROM   PRESSURE

Exercise   Splinting Positioning   Garments   Devices

Fig. 8-1. Achievement of maximum ROM and minimal scarring results in part from a program that effectively combines exercise, splinting, positioning, and pressure garments.

sure may be needed in the extremities and trunk to overcome normal capillary opening pressure.[3]

Elastic pressure wraps are used acutely until the further need for pressure is established. Each layer of elastic wrap should be applied spirally, figure of eight, or in multiple layer to produce 10 to 15 mmHg pressure. In order to achieve 20 to 40 mmHg of pressure on the trunk and the extremities, several layers are therefore indicated.[3]

Customized pressure garments are commercially available from several manufacturers. These garments must achieve at least 25 mmHg pressure and are designed to cover any area of the body in need of scar control (Fig. 8-2). Advantages of these garments include consistent pressure, less bulk and therefore less joint range of motion (ROM) restriction, ease of application, and more acceptable appearance, since the garments are worn under street clothes.

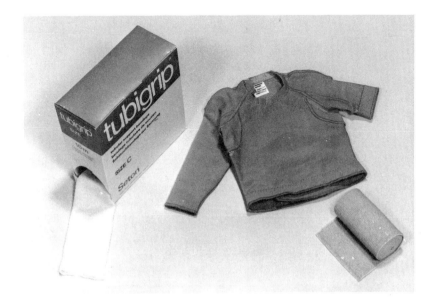

Fig. 8-2. Commercially available pressure garments and wraps.

When determining the need for pressure control, several factors must be considered. The most obvious one is the appearance of the wound. If the wound is red, edematous, itchy, and thick, it will hypertrophy and needs pressure therapy. Knowledge of the depth of the injury and the length of time elapsed before definitive wound closure is additional information that is needed. For example, if the burn was a superficial partial-thickness injury and healed in less than 10 to 14 days, the chance of hypertrophic scarring is minimal. However, if the burn invaded the dermis as a deep partial- or full-thickness injury, then the process of collagen synthesis may have been triggered. When wound closure is achieved by skin grafting, a natural form of pressure is placed over the injured tissue, which controls its growth and normalizes the structuring of these tissues.[2] Some additional pressure is generally needed to reinforce the interspaces between the grafts and interspaces where spontaneous healing occurred.

Once the need for the garments has been established, the patient is instructed to wear them continuously, removing them only for bathing purposes. "The dynamics of burn scar hypertrophy are such that interruption of pressure for eight hours may necessitate days to regain the accomplished effect."[3]

Scar tissue responds best to this pressure within the first three to six months postburn. As time between healing and the application of pressure increases, favorable results decrease. In essence, "the younger the scar, the better the response."[3]

The therapist must educate the patient on the importance of pressure application as a part of the total program for successful rehabilitation. As the vascularity of the scar tissue subsides, the patient will find a softening and increased pliability of the tissue, which allows him greater flexibility for concurrent exercise, positioning, and splinting endeavors.

Increasing Range of Motion

Limitation of motion necessitates comprehensive evaluation by the therapist. Multiple structures, in addition to the taut superficial scar, may contribute to decreased ROM. Structural limits to ROM include the underlying muscles, tendons, ligaments, joint capsule, fascia, and bone. Tightening of these structures is often an indirect result of the persistent cutaneous inflexibility. Examples of this are the formation of heterotopic bone (see Ch. 6) and the accelerated synthesis of collagen, both of which have been observed in burn patients.[5,6]

The therapist will need to identify which structures are involved and specifically stretch them. Guidelines for stretching structures are cited in several different references.[7,8]

Connective tissue displays viscoelastic properties. Tissue with such properties can be stretched or permanently deformed if forces of low intensity and long duration are applied. The use of this type of force to reduce burn scar contracture should prove to be highly successful. Desirable responses during this low-grade sustained stretch include blanching of the scar tissue across single or multiple joints and adjacent surfaces and a measurable increase in length and range of motion. Adverse responses include tearing of scar tissue or pain and edema which persist for more than two hours poststretching. These findings suggest that too much external force was applied and may result in rupture of newly formed scar tissue and blood vessels, which in turn increases scar and contracture formation.[9]

CONCEPTS AND EVALUATION OF EXERCISE-SPLINTING-POSITIONING AND PRESSURE (E-S-P-P) PROGRAM

During the rehabilitation phase, the therapist will need to reevaluate the exercises used in the acute phase and continue to include splinting, positioning, and pressure programs to keep well-ahead of active scar tissue formation and changes.

Exercise

In the initial acute stages, resistive exercise may be avoided because of the inability of the patient's cardiovascular system to adequately respond to additional stress. As wound closure is approached and completed, the patient's hypermetabolic state diminishes, and the cardiopulmonary response begins to normalize, so that additional work loads can be tolerated.[10,11]

Muscle atrophy and generalized deconditioning become evident following the long hospitalization usually associated with burn care. For the patient to effectively counteract the forces of scar tissue and prolonged inactivity, a program of graded resistive exercise should be instituted. Antagonists to the force of the contracture need to be strengthened to compete with the deforming forces of the myofibroblasts and collagen matrix. An example is the propensity of the knee to contract in flexion. The quadriceps muscle group is likely to atrophy with prolonged bedrest, and building muscle bulk in the anterior thigh as soon as possible will counteract the forces contracting the knee into flexion. A controlled, slow, smooth, sustained motion will maximize the result and reduce the unwanted stress on the new scar tissue.

Proprioceptive Neuromuscular Facilitation (PNF) techniques should be incorporated into the posthospitalization exercise program.[12] In the early phase, the component extremity patterns can be used for multiaxial range of motion and strengthening. The importance of this concept is easily seen in the patients with upper extremity and trunk burns. Elbow extension in these patients is often lost with simultaneous shoulder elevation. This reflects a lack of multiaxial joint function because of the concurrent stretcing of the linear scar tissue along the entire longitudinal axis of the extremity. To maintain suppleness of the joint structures and strengthen specific muscles when multijoint full ROM cannot be accomplished, isolated single joint motion is recommended. As a general guideline, active motion, which allows physiological joint motion and muscle action, is preferred to passive motion. However, if active motion cannot provide full excursion, then a passive stretch should be cautiously applied. These above concepts can be effected manually or with exercise equipment.

Rotational and normal timing of synergistic movements are generally non-existent in the movement patterns of burn victims. Knott and Voss propose the use of sequenced mat and extremity patterns, augmented by the therapist's manual contacts and commands, to facilitate the desired movement.[12] Mat progression and component patterns should also be used in the later stages to fine-tune visual-motion coordination and timing.

Splinting

Synthesis of collagen in burn scar does not reach its peak until four to six months post burn.[2,4] Exercise alone is often not sufficient to counteract the pull of the myofibroblasts responsible for burn scar contractures. Therefore continuation of the splinting regimen is essential to provide a second crucial counterforce designed to reduce contracture.

Splinting involves the use of controlled mechanical forces to decrease the existing deformity or to increase the ROM. When the therapist makes effective utilization of these basic concepts, all structures that interfere with joint motion, especially connective tissue, will yield to the permanent deforming forces.

In choosing which type of splinting methods to use, that is, dynamic or static, a thorough understanding of the desired outcome is essential. For example, if the goal of the splinting regimen is to increase strength of opposing muscle groups and reduce contracture, then perhaps serial splinting of an elbow flexion contracture will allow the patient to extend away from the splint while blocking unwanted flexion. In this manner, the use of the splint supplements the upgraded exercise program. Consideration of the anatomical structure to be mobilized will determine whether to utilize static or dynamic methods. Fess illustrates this by citing an example of skin contracture at the carpal metacarpal joint of the thumb which yields better results using serial web spacers to increase motion as opposed to dynamic traction at that location.[13] However, dynamic traction applied to the metacarpophalangeal (MCP) joints of the fingers for the same dysfunction is preferred to increase flexion at that location.

Determination of the amount of motion to be restored influences the splinting method chosen. An example of this is the commonly seen PIP joint flexion contracture. If the contracture measures greater than 30 degrees, a dynamic splint is used. If the proxima linterphalangeal (PIP) flexion contracture measures less than 30 degrees, a static splint will provide the necessary force to reduce the contracture.[13] Static splints can also be used to preserve attained ROM by positioning the part to keep the joints in closed pack position (Table 8-1)

Prior to fabricating the most appropriate splint for the particular problem, the therapist should evaluate the ability of the skin to tolerate additional forces, the presence of conflicting deformities, and the patient's reaction to the wearing schedule and cosmetic appearance of the splint. The therapist should also evaluate the splint itself for ease of fabrication, application, contour, and ability for functional use of adjacent nonsplinted structures.

Positioning

During rehabilitation, positioning is a necessary adjunct to the total splinting, exercise, and pressure management program. With exercise and splinting, positioning provides a third counterforce against active scar tissue contracture. The rationale for

Table 8-1. Joint Closed-Packed Positions

Joint	Position
Upper extremity	
Glenohumeral	Combined abduction and external rotation
Humeroradial	Halfway between pronation and supination
Radioulnar	
Humeroulnar	
Radiocarpal	Full extension
Intercarpal	
Interphalangeal	
Metacarpaophalangeal	Full flexion
First carpometacarpal	Full opposition
Lower extremity	
Hip	Full extension with internal rotation
Knee	Full extension with tibia externally rotated on the femur
Talocrural	Full dorsiflexion
Talar	Combined dorsiflexion and inversion

(Modified from MacConaill MA: Joint movement. Physiotherapy 50:363, 1964)

utilization of positioning is the same as that presented in previous discussion. In addition to the previous program, the patient should be instructed to be conscious of alternate ways to incorporate positioning into his daily routine.

Areas that are difficult to splint may be stretched more effectively by positioning. For instance, placing the patient with a neck burn on staggered double mattresses with the neck positioned above the first mattress in hyperextension maximizes stretch of the scar tissue while effectively utilizing rest periods (Fig. 8-3).

Another area that is usually difficult to splint, but which positions nicely and utilizes gravity is the anterior chest. If towel rolls are arranged parallel to the spine beneath the supine patient, a slow gentle retraction of the shoulders will ensue, with gentle stretching of the upper anterior chest scar tissue.

Positioning can be combined with gentle forces in addition to gravity. A commonly used position to stretch knee flexion contractures is to place the patient prone, add a velcro cuff weight to the ankle, and ask the patient to actively extend the knee. If the knee is serially splinted, all three counterforces—exercise, splinting, and positioning—are utilized.

Evaluation of E-S-P-P Program

Effective application and evaluation of the concepts of E-S-P-P will make the burn team's goals of minimizing scarring and contracture more attainable. When evaluating the components of the total program, the key points discussed in the following pages should be noted.

Exercise. Factors that indicate appropriate choice and implementation of elements of the exercise regimen include:

Increased ROM   The therapist should keep records of standard goniometric measurements for both single axis and multiple axis joint actions. If there is a limitation of the ROM, identify the structure limits and modify the program to affect them.

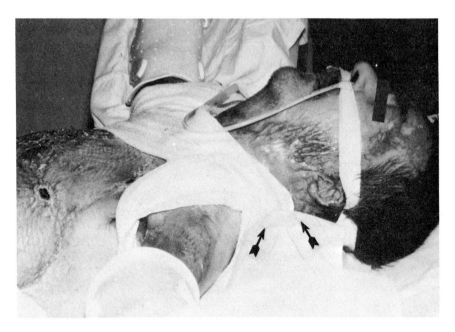

Fig. 8-3. Hyperextension of the neck on double mattresses for stretch of anterior neck and trunk scar tissue.

Because multiple joints and support structures may be involved in the injury of the burned hand, goniometric records of isolated joint motions do not effectively evaluate the actual tissue involvment. Utilization of the total active movement (TAM) rating scale has its advantages, as it establishes a scale that rates the combined motion or lack of it for the entire digit (Table 8-2).

Increased Muscle Strength and Endurance. The therapist should record results of regular manual muscle tests or isotonic/isokinetic recordings, which can substantiate the program's effectiveness.

Observance of Gait Pattern. The therapist should observe the patient's pattern of gait or rotational components, normal timing, and postural habits. Joint restrictions and muscle weakness problems that lead to gait irregularities will often initially manifest themselves in these observations.

Total Body Conditioning. Total body conditioning will become evident as the patient's postdischarge activity level increases. Cardiopulmonary endurance is checked by recording vital signs before and after exercising against a fixed work load, or by asking the patient to keep a diary of daily activities and responses.

Table 8-2. Total Active Motion (TAM) Rating Scale

Normal	260°
Excellent	220°–259°
Good	180°–219°
Poor	180°–less

Improvement in all four preceding areas should appear after several weeks. The successful result of any exercise program depends on routine compliance. For many patients and their families, coping with the ordeals of postdischarge lifestyle is overwhelming, and exercise programs may be ignored. The therapist may select from several methods to reestablish patient cooperation. One method would be to regain closer supervision of the patient's exercise routine by increasing the frequency of outpatient visits and/or by enlisting the help of other health care team members for home visits. Another approach would be to simplify the program so that the patient is able to duplicate it at home.

If the patient becomes involved in establishing short- and long-term goals, participation in the total program will improve. Occasionally, the therapist will encounter the patient for whom none of the preceding interventions work. Behavioral contracting may be the only way to handle a totally noncompliant patient.[14]

Often times, the exercise program is too cumbersome, especially with a large percent of skin involvement. Either the patient fatigues before completion or states that he doesn't have sufficient time during the day to devote to an extensive exercise program. In this case, the splinting, positioning, and pressure components of the program must be strengthened.

Splinting. The therapist will need to periodically reevaluate the effectiveness of the splinting program to assure that it is functioning in coordination with the goals of the exercise-positioning-pressure programs. Frequent passive and active ROM measurements will supply the therapist with standard objective measurements.

As physical changes occur, appropriate changes in the mechanical force exerted by the splint will need to be made. Daily modifications of the splint may be required when serial splinting is applied. Some adverse effects of splinting to be watched for include skin irritation and breakdown, neurovascular symptoms, and edema and pain that persist after the initial wearing session. Signs of a successful splinting program include the absence of adverse responses, reduction of contracture, and increased range of motion.

Pressure. Signs that the pressure program has been successful can be seen as early as 24 to 48 hours after the initial application. Immediately after the removal of the garment, evidence of clinically significant pressure includes blanching of scar tissue, flattening of the scar, increased softness, decreased edema, minimal blistering, and no complaints of neurovascular impairment, that is, tingling or numbness. If any of these effects are not observed, the therapist should consider the following reasons:

Fit of garment: If the patient has gained or lost over ten pounds, this may be enough to decrease the pressure garment's effectiveness;[15]

Condition of a garment: The wear life of pressure garments for the average patient is three months. If the garment loses its stretch and doesn't cause blanching of the scar, it has lost its effectiveness and new garments must be made.

Some scar tissue breakdown is to be expected. High risk areas, such as posterior aspect of the elbow, axillary folds, popliteal and antecubital space, web spaces, and joints of the fingers and toes, can be somewhat protected by padding pressure points to increase distribution of the pressure.

When isolated areas of hypertrophy remain, significant pressure has not been applied. Areas where this commonly occurs include the sternum, face, volar aspect of the hand, angle of the mandible, web spaces, and across the flex surfaces of the joint. Pressure garments frequently need to be supplemented by inserts in these areas in order to exert the needed pressure. Consideration of the area of the body being treated, skin mobility, and anatomical contour all must be considered when ordering pressure garments. Once these factors are known, appropriate pressure inserts are selected. Characteristics to be considered in choosing the composition of the insert include its texture, flexibility, compressibility, and ability to conform.[16]

As scar tissue approaches maturity, the hyperemia fades and the scar flattens and becomes more pliable and soft. When these qualities persist for several weeks after removal of the pressure garments, the scar tissues is mature, and the garments may be discontinued.

SPECIAL CONSIDERATIONS

Face

Complex topographical contour organs of special sensation and the balance between the myofascial-cutaneous interfaces all present special problems in the control of scarring and contracture in this area. Distortion of facial symmetry can result in a very disfigured appearance.

The principles of exercise, especially those advocated by Knott and Voss, optimally take advantage of the intimacy of facial musculature to its overlying skin.[12]

Microstomia, or loss of vertical and horizontal dimensions of the mouth, is both a cosmetically unpleasant and functionally inhibiting complication of perioral burns. A patient with such a deformity cannot eat properly or perform adequate oral hygiene, and presents special problems regarding surgical corrective procedures.[17] Several types of microstomia mouth conformer devices can be readily fabricated or purchased prefabricated. These devices apply static or dynamic pressures to the corners of the mouth, cheeks, and mucosal linings to counteract the pull of scar tissue. They are, however, extremely awkward to wear and require constant adjustment and inspection by the therapist.

There are several different methods available for providing adequate pressure over highly contoured facial areas. The customized elastic face mask generally needs to be supplemented with inserts fabricated of silicone or thermoplastics to produce optimal pressure on facial contours. Transparent face masks designed by Rivers offer an alternative to the mask appearance of an elastic garment.[18] Transparent high temperature plastic gives the patient a more pleasing appearance, is custom made to give greater pressure, and allows visual access for evaluation.[18]

Neck

The predisposition of the neck to form postburn flexion contractures poses special problems for exercise, splinting, and pressure regimens. Devices such as the thermoplastic conformer splint and the transparent polyvinyl chloride (PVC) neck orthosis immobilize the mandible, position the cervical spine in hyperextension, and provide sufficient contact for scar control.[19]

These devices do not, however, allow rotational or lateral movement of the cervical spine. The Watusi neck splint, which is composed of stacks of closed cell cylindrical pads, is less rigid and allows for these additional movements while limiting cervical flexion and applying constant pressure.[20]

A program that alternates combinations of these appliances described above may offer a compromise solution.

Positioning during rest periods and nighttime on double-stacked staggered mattresses places the cervical spine in hyperextension for a prolonged stretch to the anterior neck and chest scar. The patient should also be instructed to assume beneficial postural positions while participating in activities of daily living (ADL).

Neck exercise programs require the removal of splints, but nevertheless should be performed routinely in combination with facial and upper chest exercises to indicate multiaxial movement and stretch. However, even with a well-supervised program and a cooperative patient, the presence of significant neck contracture following moderate to severe thermal trauma to the anterior neck is not uncommon.

Trunk

The surface area of the trunk represents 36 percent of the total body surface area. Postural and gait problems and hypertrophic scarring are common problems seen after significant burn injury to this large and commonly injured area.

Kyphosis, lordosis, or a combination of the two is frequently seen in adult trunk burns from the active pull of scar tissue. Severe scar contracture of the skin and trunk or groin in children may result in scoliotic curvature of the spine.[21] These conditions can be identified early if the therapist is continually vigilant for the possibility of postural problems. General postural and scoliosis exercises that will strengthen antagonist muscles and stretch the agonist muscles are essential and may prove useful in those patients who seem, by the nature of their injuries, to be particularly prone to develop this deformity.

Utilization of several splinting devices in conjunction with postural exercise programs may be necessary in cases of severe postural deviation. Becker has fabricated a device that retracts the shoulders, extends the cervical and thoracic spine, and also provides pressure to difficult areas.[22] Clavicular slings or figure of eight Ace wrappings around the shoulders apply sufficient force to retract the shoulders and apply stretch to the pectoral region to counteract kyphotic tendencies.

The specialized topography of the trunk creates problems in the effective fitting of pressure garments. The bony prominence of the shoulder, clavicle, sternum, ribs, and iliac crest coupled with the soft breast projections create complex contours, which seem to defy the application of adequate pressure. Inserts designed to fill the void between the garment and the scar may be necessary. One method of securing inserts to the trunk is to prepare a garment with custom-fitted inserts attached. When fashioning such a device, have the patient wear a snug-fitting undershirt and apply the silicone elastomer directly to the contour area. Allow the elastomer to penetrate the shirt and set. The custom-fabricated inserts will then be securely attached to the undershirt. In this way, the patient has only to don the undershirt to secure insert placement prior to application of the pressure vest. In order to maintain sufficient pressure, these inserts will need to be reinforced as the scar flattens.

Axilla

Webbing of scar tissue bands spanning the anterior and posterior axillary folds create limitations in ROM and significant cosmetic deformities. Because of the difficulty in applying successful pressure to the axillary folds, a combination of pressure and splinting may be required. An axillary conformer, or airplane splint, fabricated from thermoplastic material, abducts the shoulder and prolongs the stretch of the axillary webs. These splints are also used to maintain the axilla in an abducted position after surgical releases of axillary contractures.

Crescent-shaped pieces of closed-packed foam placed under the axillae and figure of eight wrapped around the shoulders and back, or the use of the clavicular sling, will apply pressure and stretch to the axillae. These devices can be worn over pressure garments. Care must be taken to observe for excessive pressure, which may cause brachial plexis irritation.

Hands

Documentation of the numerous postburn injury deformities of the hand and theraputic plans for management of such injuries is extensive.[23-26] The Boutonnière deformity of the PIP joint, the claw hand, and intrinsic-minus deformities are among the most common.

Application of pressure to control scarring and edema should be instituted soon after wound closure. Proper fitting customized pressure gloves supply adequate pressure to the digits. Areas that frequently need to be supplemented are the web spaces and the dorsum and volar aspects of the hand. Partial- and full-thickness hand burn injuries may result in loss of contour and shape of the web spaces. Loss of the dorsal slant of the web space with contraction of scar tissue supports MCP hyperextension and creates volar pockets, which present cosmetic and hygenic problems.

Juan et al. suggests the use of graded pressure inserts for control of burn syndactyly. The selection of the insert depends upon the patient's skin tolerance to pressure. As tolerance increases, the inserts may be designed to be more compressive. Inserts may be designed to be worn either inside or outside the glove. (Fig. 8-4).[27] A survey of this technique indicates that less surgical intervention was necessary with the use of pressure graded insert programs.

Dorsal scarring can be easily controlled by inserts of silicone, elastomer, or dense foam placed under the pressure glove. Donut-shaped mole-skin pads stacked and placed over bony prominences will redistribute adverse pressure exerted by the glove. Volar scar tissue contraction, although rare, results in abduction of the thenar and hypothenar eminences with loss of the intereminence concavity. Thermoplastic inserts that produce a consistent pressure may be helpful in preventing this deformity. Careful fit of these inserts will allow the patient active functional use of the hand.

Knee and Elbow

Control and management of burn scars of the antecubital and popliteal areas are similar, since both are prone to hypertrophic scar, flexion contracture, and frequent breakdown.

Posthospitalization continuation of the therapeutic plan initiated in the hospital may be sufficient to prevent further deformities in these areas. However, the tendency toward contracture is high, and additional measures, such as surgical release, may be necessary.[28] If contracture develops early, fabrication of contour serial splints applied to the antecubital and popliteal areas and combined with active extension away from the splint will reduce these contractures. The splints may require daily reshaping. When full extension is achieved, three point elbow or knee splints are substituted.[3] Night wear of the conformer splints, avoidance of long sessions of sitting with knees flexed, and progressive resistive exercise (PRE) to quadriceps will maintain knee extension.

Pressure garments used in these areas tend to bind and irritate, especially in the presence of contracture bands. The use of soft padding inserts over these areas will eliminate this nuisance and potential breakdown point.

Ankle and Foot

Potential problems of the foot and ankle include hyperextension of the toes, subluxation of the metatarsals and plantar flexion-inversion restrictions. To stretch the scar tissue that restricts plantar flexion, the use of night splints across the dorsum of the foot and ankle allow optimal stretch. Daytime wear of high-topped orthopedic shoes that have long tongues padded with one-half-inch felt supplements the night splint regime.

Tightness of the scar across the dorsum of the foot produces hyperextension of the toes and, in extreme cases, subluxation of the metatarsal heads. Nothdurft et al. suggest preventative treatment by using flexion wraps to the toes combined with counterpressure against the metatarsal heads provided by a thermoplastic soleplate. In preexisting subluxation, addition of a metatarsal bar to the orthopedic high-topped shoes adds a counterforce to combat the active dorsal stretch provided by the shoe.[29] Both the patient and the therapist must be aware of early signs of breakdown on the dorsum of the foot and toes.

Extra depth shoes available at most orthopedic specialty shops provide extra space. Plastizote inserts to counteract metatarsal subluxation tendencies can be fashioned into the shoe and are often more cosmetically acceptable to the patient (Fig. 8-5). Layers of moleskin pressure relief (bunion) pads can be used across toe joints to redistribute pressure around the joint. In addition, customized elastic garments with

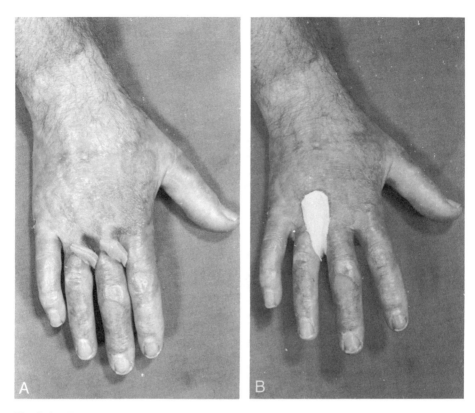

Fig. 8-4. Pressure-graded inserts to wear under pressure glove for control of syndactyly. (A) soft foam, (B) silicone elastomer.

enclosed toes will hold foam or Silastic inserts in proper position. Addition of one or two cotton or wool socks decreases frictional forces and absorbs moisture.

Gait

As mentioned in Chapter 4, gait normalization is part of the acute therapy plan, but must be refined in the postdischarge plan. Waiting until the patient is free from contracture and painful areas of skin breakdown does not automatically result in a smooth, rhythmic gait. Posthospitalization additions of awkward pressure garments, devices, and splints is often enough to discourage most patients from resuming a normal preinjury gait.

The subleties and complexities of a smooth-flowing gait must be analyzed by the therapist from many different perspectives. Use of mirrors, metronomes, and pressure sensitive paper are a few of the methods available to provide the patient with the feedback necessary to correct for months of habitual guarding and the new feel of his scarred body.

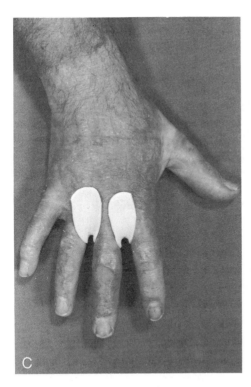 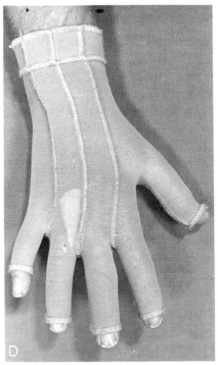

Fig. 8-4 (*Continued*). (C) low temperature plastic, and (D) glove over insert.

MODALITIES

Paraffin

"Scarring, with the loss of elasticity and excessive dryness, leads to decreased motion, which, in turn may partially or completely immobilize the joint, resulting in tightness and pain within the joint itself."[30] As more aggressive measures are instituted after discharge, cracking and breakdown of the scar tissue often occurs. Lubrication of these areas with creams and lotions does not provide prolonged relief or ease the pain of mobilization of tight joints. The use of the paraffin bath has been promoted for relaxation of skeletal muscle spasm. Head and Helm emphasize that paraffin also lubricates and increases the extensibility of the collagen tissues in burn scars. The paraffin mixture is used when it reaches a temperature of 46° to 48°C, or when a light skim covers the top of the mixture. Head and Helm suggest the addition of 2.5 ounces of oil to each pound of paraffin, thereby reducing its melting point to approximately 39°C.[30] Caution is suggested for newly healed scar tissue, which will blister easily if the standard paraffin bath temperature is used.

Pouring or patting of the paraffin is done after the patient is positioned with the

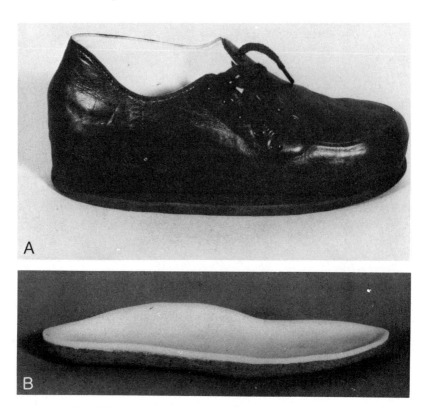

Fig. 8-5.   (A) Extra depth shoes and (B) Platizote insert.

affected part in a sustained maximum stretch and wrapped with cellophane and toweling. The treatment time is 20 to 30 minutes. Patients report decreased joint pain, and objective measurements showed a five to ten degree increase in ROM after paraffin treatment. Claims that the results last up to four hours were documented. With proper instruction, this routine can be an appropriate adjunct to the patient's home program.

Ultrasound

Several investigators cite the usefulness of ultrasound in the treatment of burn scars.[31-33] Others maintain that favorable results are obtained only in the presence of hypertophic scarring and not in the presence of keloids.

The physiological effects attributed to ultrasound include the elevation of tissue temperature to increase the extensibility of the disorganized collagen, decrease of the viscosity of the collagen ground substance, and increase in pain threshold.[35] The use of mineral oil as the coupling agent during ultrasound treatments also lubricates dry skin. Frequent application of mineral oil will be necessary as direct contact with the ultrasound head liquefies the couplant.[35]

Whirlpools

Several centers have found the use of the whirlpool for exercise as a valuable adjunct to the posthospital period. However, posthospitalization use of whirlpools for exercise during this period appears to have less desirable results. Intentions of gaining a generalized heating effect with submersion may result in edema, itching, and the dissipation of natural skin lubricants. Some patients also complain of "rebound" stiffness.

Massage

Benefits from massage include reduction in edema and manual assistance to lymphatic function. In addition, the direct human contact is soothing to the patient. The patient's skin is gradually more tolerant of massage as the posthospitalization period progresses.

A deep-kneading massage technique should be chosen, as this decreases the friction transmitted through the superficial skin layers. To enhance firmer contact, lotion should not be used during massage. Blanching of the tissues is a favorable indication that adequate massage has been applied. A very light effleurage with a lotion should follow to lubricate the skin and increase venous and lymphatic flow.[36]

The above regimen is administered twice daily. With proper instruction, the patient and his family can incorporate this procedure into a home program.

SKIN CARE

As discharge from hospital approaches, precautions and instructions for skin care are given to the patient and his family. However, once the patient leaves the hospital, he encounters new situations and will seek answers from the most available person. Frequently, this person is the therapist who continues to observe the patient during his daily or weekly outpatient visits.

Breakdown and Blistering

Areas of skin breakdown, blistering, or chronic granulation tissue frequently persist for three to six months postburn. These areas are commonly found over joints or areas where clothing, splints, and other objects cause repeated trauma. The therapist must prevent these areas of breakdown by identifying and eliminating potential sources of trauma. The use of nonadherent dressings and wraps inserted between pressure garments and splints buffers the frictional forces transmitted to the skin. Frequent adjustments of splints reduces unwanted areas of pressure and ischemia. Perspiration under splints and clothing may cause maceration to the fragile skin. Frequent change of clothes, use of nonirritating antiperspirants, drying the moisture from the splint, and a light dusting with baby powder or cornstarch will absorb some of the excess moisture. Overzealous stretching and cracking of scar tissue during exercise may also cause chronic irritation. Appropriate application of moisturizers aid dry, cracking skin.

Protective sensation in burned and grafted areas will be diminished in relation to destruction of the underlying sensory receptors. These receptors are housed in the corium and may be partially or completely destroyed depending upon the depth of the burn. Areas of thick hypertrophic tissue and donor areas will vary in their receptive characteristics. Focusing the patient's attention on this deficit may lessen unhealthy breakdown from frictional forces and promote avoidance of potentially harmful situations.

Small areas of breakdown, if appropriately treated, do not delay the wearing of pressure garments. In addition, reassurance to the patient that this is a frequent occurrence eases his fear of rehospitalization for skin coverage.

Lotions and Creams

The patient finds frequent skin lubrication beneficial in the posthospitalization period. Sebaceous glands, if not totally destroyed, will reestablish function 2 to 18 months postburn.[37]

Selection of an appropriate lubricant involves choosing a lotion that is mild, nonirritating, and yields the most relief from itching and dryness. Many such lotions and creams are available. The patient should be instructed to select the product that produces the best results for him. As the characteristics of scar tissue change, so does the choice of lubricant.

The patient is instructed to apply the lubricant frequently in minimal amounts. The use of effleurage massage to disperse the lotion and the removal of excess amounts prior to application of pressure garments helps avoid skin maceration.

Sunscreens

The newly healed skin is deficient in protective pigment and is highly sensitive to ultraviolet rays of the sun.[37] The recently discharged patient is instructed to avoid all direct sun exposure. In order to avoid unwanted discoloration and blistering of the new delicate skin, the patient wears protective clothing and hats. The patient should select times when the sun's rays are minimal for outdoor exposure.

Use of commercial sunscreen is important to protect the newly healed skin that is not covered by clothing. Many products are available and selection is based on the patient's requirements. Some products will remain on the skin after swimming or perspiration, whereas others require reapplication after such activities. A few moisture creams contain sunscreen, so it is wise to read the product literature before purchasing. Generally, one or two years postburn, activities in full sun can be resumed.

Itching

Stimulation of nerve endings facilitates the urge to itch. Of all of the postburn problems, patients frequently complain of itching most bitterly. Proper lubrication of the skin, wearing of pressure garments, and use of mild bath soap all lessen this state of urgency. Activities and temperatures that initiate perspiration are reported to decrease itching.

The physician may also prescribe oral antihistamines and topical corticosteroid creams to offer the patient some temporary relief. Itching generally subsides as the pliability of the scar tissue progresses.

Thermoregulation

Full integrity of the skin and dermal appendages is required to dissipate heat. In deep partial- and full-thickness burns, thermoregulation is impaired. Decreased vascularity and reduced sweat mechanisms in the scar tissue combine to diminish the efficiency of the body's ability to dissipate heat. In 30 percent of patients studied in Ben-Simchon's research with 20 to 60 percent total burn surface areas, their thermoregulatory abilities were impaired.[38] Palmer et al. declare that patients with major burns are ". . . physiologically handicapped in cold exposure." Their research illustrated that patients who were 1½ to 10 years postburn did not tolerate cold temperatures as well as a comparable group of unburned patients. The study concluded that there was an increased vasomotor response of blood vessels of a skin graft and scar tissue, which increased metabolic heat production while core temperature remained unchanged.[39]

Members of the burn team will hear multiple complaints from patients concerning their intolerance to heat and cold. The team members can educate the patient about thermoregulatory impairment and advise them to make modifications in lifestyle in order to avoid potentially harmful situations. Education as to the signs and symptoms of temperature intolerance, modification of stressful activity in heat, and the avoidance of prolonged exposure to the cold is helpful. The staff can also help the patient in the proper selection of clothing, such as lightweight, loose cotton garments in the summer and multiple layers in the winter.

Cosmetics

The introduction of cosmetics is a relatively new concept to be included in the final phase of rehabilitation. Clear definition concerning which burn team member should present this information varies from center to center.

When the physician deems the patient's scars as mature and has recommended discontinuation of the pressure garments, application of cosmetics can be initiated. It is usually at this time that the patient's feeling of an unsatisfactory final appearance is manifested. Some patients may not want to reveal the uneven tone and texture of their skin and may seek to continue to wear postburn compression garments in an effort to disguise their appearance. Others may find themselves unemployable because of their new appearance. Studies by Bowden and Feller have shown that women use the image of self and body as a source of self-esteem, whereas men's self-esteem correlates more with employment status.[40]

Care must be taken to educate patients in the appropriate selection and use of cosmetics. Many patients find that their preburn cosmetic and method of application is no longer suitable for several reasons:

The makeup is not absorbed because of absence or distortion of skin pores.
Areas of color mismatch or depigmentation in proximity to the more even-toned skin.
Absence or distortion of facial features result in asymetrical appearance.[41]

Given the proper information, the patient can gain self-confidence and create a more satisfying appearance with the proper use of cosmetics.

PSYCHOSOCIAL POSTDISCHARGE PROBLEMS

Discharge from the sheltered environment of the hospital often creates another crisis for the patient and family. Not only will a myriad of physical changes continue to plague the patient, but also confrontation with emotional reactions and interactions will surface. Various authors have identified the first 12 months after the injury as the postburn mourning period.[42]

Andreasen details numerous psychological traits that these patients display. These traits include separation anxiety, traumatic and phobic neuroses, and grief. He states that these complex feelings are often manifested in frequent crying spells, insomnia, anxiety, fear of fire or circumstances that are reminiscent of the incident, and sudden realization of the loss of family, home, and financial security. Andreasen concurs with most authors that these reactions and emotions peak during the first year postinjury and regress as the years progress.[43]

Of all the burn team members, the physical therapist often has the most frequent contact with patients during this postburn period. Many patients are eager to discuss their emotions and inabilities to cope with them; others are not. By being sensitive to what is always a difficult adjustment, the therapist can facilitate this adjustment and recognize the need for the skills of other team members, such as psychiatrists, psychologists, or social workers. Behavior that may signal a change in the patient's ability to cope may be reflected in his lack of compliance with the program, failure to keep scheduled appointments, and unrealistic expectations concerning physical appearance and functional abilities.

Many different factors contribute to the rebuilding of feelings of self-worth and self-image. The support of family and friends and society has been documented as the most important strength upon which the patient draws.[44] Attainment of established goals in therapy can be one way to support the patient's development of self-esteem. "Most new self-esteem is based on their demonstrated ability to triumph over external limitations."[43] The posthospitalization phase is a period of adjustment for the patient and his family. A successful plan for rehabilitation must then be based on a comprehensive view of the patient psychologically, socially, and physically.[42]

ACKNOWLEDGEMENT

Sincere appreciation to Mary T. Perlstein, RPT, who fostered my professional growth and endeavors in the treatment of burn victims.

REFERENCES

1. Gordon: Role of the discharge planning and outpatient clinic nurse. J of Burn Care Rehab 1:31, 1981
2. Larson DL, Huang T, Dobrkovsky M, Baur PS, Parks DH: Prevention and treatment of scar contracture. In: Burns—A Team Approach, eds. Artz CP, Moncrief JA, Pruit B. Philadelphia, WB Saunders, 1979
3. Parks H, Baur PS, Larson DL: Late problems in burns. Clin Plast Surg 4:547, 1977
4. Larson DL: Contracture and scar formation in the burn patient. Clin Plast Surg 4:653, 1974
5. Evans EB, Larson DL, Yates S: Preservation and restoration of joint function in patients with severe burns. JAMA 204:91, 1968
6. Peacock, EE: Some biochemical and biophysical aspects of joint stiffness: role of collagen synthesis as opposed to altered molecular bonding. Annals of Surg 164:1, 1966
7. Beaulieu J: Developing a stretching program. Physician and Sports Medicine 9:59, 1981
8. Sapega A: Biophysical factors in ROM exercises. Physician and Sports Medicine 9:51, 1981
9. Edstem LE, Robson MC, Headley BT: Evaluation of exercise techniques in the burn patient. Burns 4:113, 1981
10. Black S, Carter GM, Nitz AJ, Worthington JA: Oxygen consumption for lower extremity exercises in normal subjects and burn patients. Phys Ther 60:1255, 1980
11. Wilmore DW: Nutrition and metabolism following thermal injury. Clin Plast Surg 1:603, 1974
12. Knott M, Voss DE: Propioceptive Neuromuscular Facilitation. New York, Harper and Row, 1968
13. Fess E, Gettle K, Strickland J: Hand splinting principles and methods. St. Louis, CV Mosby, 1981
14. Simons RD, McFadd A, Frank HA: Behavioral contracting in a burn care facility: a strategy for patient participation. J Trauma 18:257 1978
15. Jobst Institute: Answering your questions about Burnscar and Jōbskin™ custom-made pressure covers. Toledo Jobst Institute, 1979
16. Alston DW, Kozerefski P: Materials for pressure inserts in the control of hypertrophic scars. Journal Burn Care Rehabilitation 2:40, 1981
17. Clark WR, McDade GO: Microstomia in burn victims: a new appliance for prevention and treatment and literature review. Journal Burn Care and Rehabilitation 1:33, 1980
18. Rivers EA, Strate RG, Solem LD: The transparent face mask. AJOT 33:108, 1979
19. Feldman AE, MacMillan BG: Burn injury in children: declining need for reconstructive surgery as related to use of neck orthoses. Arch Phys Med Rehab 61:441, 1980
20. Sandel E, Khahecli CR: Use of thermoplastic total contact and the foam Watusi ring neck splints. American O.T. Assoc. Newsletter, 4 1981
21. Artz CP, Moncrief JA: The treatment of burns. Philadelphia, WB Saunders, 1969

22. Becker BE: Hypertrophic burn scarring: control of chest deformities with a new device. Arch Phys Med Rehab 61:187, 1980
23. Salisbury RE, Pruitt BA: Burns of the upper extremity. Philadelphia, WB Saunders, 1976
24. Malick MA: Manual on Dynamic Splinting with Thermoplastic Materials. Pittsburgh, Harmarville Rehabilitation Center, 1974
25. Hunter JM, Schneider LH, Mackin EJ, Bell JA: Rehabilitation of the Hand. St. Louis, CV Mosby, 1978
26. Weeks PM, Wray CR: Management of Acute Hand Injuries a Biological Approach. St. Louis, CV Mosby, 1978
27. Quan PE, Rau SB, Alston DW: Control of scar tissue in finger web spaces by use of graded pressure inserts. Journal of Burn Care and Rehabilitation 1:27, 1980
28. Dobbs ER, Curreri WP: Burns: analysis of results of physical therapy in 681 patients. J Trauma 12:242, 1972
29. Nothdurft D, Pullium G, Bruster J: Management of feet and ankle burns: orthotic management of preexisting deformity and protocol for prevention of deformity. Burns 5:221, 1979
30. Head MD, Helm PA: Paraffin and sustained stretching in the treatment of burn contracture. Burns 4:136, 1978
31. Rozanova EP: The use of ultrasonics for the prevention of contractures after burns. Orthopedia Traumatolgiia 34:13, 1979
32. Belenger M, VanderElst E, Toussaint JP: New contributions to treatment of localized burns of the hand. Ann Chir Plast 9:199, 1969
33. Faure J, Vanden Bulcke L: Ultrasonic treatment of burns. J Belge Rheu Med Phys 20:239, 1965
34. Wright ET, Haase KH: Keloids and Ultrasound. Arch Phys Med Rehab 52:280, 1971
35. Griffin JE, Karseilis TC: Ultrasonic energy. In: Physical Agents for Physical Therapists. Springfield, Charles C. Thomas, 1978
36. Tappan FM: Effects of massage. In: Healing Massage Techniques A Study of Eastern and Western Methods. Reston Publishing Company, Inc., Reston, 1978
37. Trotter M, Johnson CS: The Treatment of Burn Patients A Study Manual for Physical Therapists. Health Sciences Learning Resources Center and Division of Physical Therapy, University of Washington, 1979
38. Ben-Simchon C, Tsur H: Heat intolerance in patients with extensive healed burns. Pl Reconstr Surg 6:499, 1981
39. Palmer B, Jacobsson S, Malm L: Patients with healed major burns in hot and cold environments. Burns 5:79, 1978
40. Bowden ML, Feller I: Self-esteem of severly burned patients. Arch Phys Med Rehab 61:449, 1980
41. Salisbury F: Cosmetics for the burn patient: the illusion of reality. Abstract American Burn Association Mtg, Washington, 1981
42. Blades B, Jones C, Munster AM: Quality of life after major burns. J Trauma 19:556, 1979
43. Andreasen NSC, Norris AS: Long-term adjustment and adaption mechanisms in severly burned adults. J Nerv Mentl Disease 154:352, 1972
44. Davidson TN, Bowden ML: Social support and postburn adjustment. Arch Phys Med Rehab 62:275, 1981

Index